Intensive Care: Clinical Principles and Practice

Intensive Care: Clinical Principles and Practice

Edited by Damien Newman

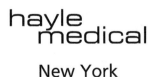

New York

Hayle Medical,
750 Third Avenue, 9th Floor,
New York, NY 10017, USA

Visit us on the World Wide Web at:
www.haylemedical.com

© Hayle Medical, 2019

This book contains information obtained from authentic and highly regarded sources. Copyright for all individual chapters remain with the respective authors as indicated. All chapters are published with permission under the Creative Commons Attribution License or equivalent. A wide variety of references are listed. Permission and sources are indicated; for detailed attributions, please refer to the permissions page and list of contributors. Reasonable efforts have been made to publish reliable data and information, but the authors, editors and publisher cannot assume any responsibility for the validity of all materials or the consequences of their use.

ISBN: 978-1-63241-592-9

Trademark Notice: Registered trademark of products or corporate names are used only for explanation and identification without intent to infringe.

Cataloging-in-Publication Data

    Intensive care : clinical principles and practice / edited by Damien Newman.
       p. cm.
    Includes bibliographical references and index.
    ISBN 978-1-63241-592-9
    1. Critical care medicine. 2. Emergency medicine.
    3. Intensive care units. I. Newman, Damien.
RC86.7 .I58 2019
616.025--dc23

Table of Contents

Preface VII

Chapter 1 **Important Issues in Coma and Neuromonitoring** 1
Bogdan Pavel

Chapter 2 **Sepsis in Children** 22
Selim Öncel

Chapter 3 **Infections and Multidrug-Resistant Pathogens in ICU Patients** 48
Muntean Delia and Licker Monica

Chapter 4 **Acute Kidney Injury in the Intensive Care Unit** 69
Jose J. Zaragoza and Faustino J. Renteria

Chapter 5 **Measuring and Managing Fluid Overload in Pediatric Intensive Care Unit** 83
Dyah Kanya Wati

Chapter 6 **Intra-Abdominal Pressure Monitoring** 93
Zsolt Bodnar

Chapter 7 **Endotracheal Intubation in Children: Practice Recommendations, Insights and Future Directions** 105
Maribel Ibarra-Sarlat, Eduardo Terrones-Vargas,
Lizett Romero-Espinoza, Graciela Castañeda-Muciño,
Alejandro Herrera-Landero and Juan Carlos Núñez-Enríquez

Chapter 8 **Airway Management in ICU Settings** 128
Nabil Abdelhamid Shallik, Mamdouh Almustafa,
Ahmed Zaghw and Abbas Moustafa

Chapter 9 **Brain Death in Children** 160
Eleni Athanasios Volakli, Peristera-Eleni Mantzafleri,
Serafeia Kalamitsou, Asimina Violaki, Elpis Chochliourou,
Menelaos Svirkos, Athanasios Kasimis and Maria Sdougka

Permissions

List of Contributors

Index

Preface

Every book is initially just a concept; it takes months of research and hard work to give it the final shape in which the readers receive it. In its early stages, this book also went through rigorous reviewing. The notable contributions made by experts from across the globe were first molded into patterned chapters and then arranged in a sensibly sequential manner to bring out the best results.

Intensive care is the care of extremely ill patients who are struggling with severe and life-threatening illnesses. Such patients require constant attention, proper care, support from special equipments, and medications to be able to perform normal bodily functions. Trauma, sepsis, acute respiratory distress syndrome (ARDS) and multiple organ failure are some of the common medical conditions which are treated in an intensive care unit. Analgesics, medically induced comas and induced sedation are strategies for the management of pain and prevention of secondary infections. Some of the equipment available in an intensive care unit are hemofiltration equipment, mechanical ventilation, nasogastric tubes, catheters, drains and suction pumps. This book brings forth some of the most innovative concepts and elucidates the unexplored aspects of intensive care. The topics included herein are of utmost significance and bound to provide incredible insights to readers. The book is appropriate for students seeking detailed information in this area as well as for doctors and experts.

It has been my immense pleasure to be a part of this project and to contribute my years of learning in such a meaningful form. I would like to take this opportunity to thank all the people who have been associated with the completion of this book at any step.

Editor

Important Issues in Coma and Neuromonitoring

Bogdan Pavel

Abstract

Coma is defined as a state of unconsciousness and lack of response to noxious stimuli. The physiopathology of consciousness and coma is not entirely understood. On the other hand, clinical examination does not give us enough information in all types of coma states. In this chapter, some types of coma and their definition, the necessity of coma monitoring and what we can use for coma monitoring in ICU, algorithms for EEG monitoring, BIS, AppEntropy, permutation entropy and auditory evoked potentials are described. Burst suppression state new theories and cortical connectivity and reactivity during coma as a tool for coma prognosis will be on focus.

Keywords: coma status, burst suppression, cortical connectivity, cortical reactivity

1. Introduction

Coma is defined as a state of loss of consciousness and lack of response to external stimuli that occurs in pathological states and during anesthesia. The prognosis of coma patients is difficult to assess, as the mechanism through which coma occurs is not entirely understood. What we may do is evaluate cerebral function, through accurate and careful monitoring. Thus, the intensive care specialist requires one or several instruments to monitor the cerebral function of coma patients, as it is difficult to perform, even hourly, a clinical evaluation, taking into account the typical workload of the doctor.

In certain circumstances, a worsening neurological state does not manifest itself clinically — an example being nonconvulsive status, which has negative prognostic value in the case of traumatic brain injury (TBI), and can only be diagnosed through continuous electroencephalographic monitoring (EEG).

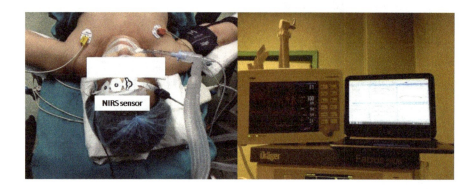

Figure 1. Continuous BIS (bispectral index) and NIRS (near-infrared spectroscopy) monitoring during anesthesia.

Continuous EEG monitoring and cerebral oximetry monitoring—through the NIRS (near-infrared spectroscopy) technique—are useful instruments that provide the doctor with real-time, vital information on the coma patient. These techniques have the advantage of noninvasivity, ease of use and they can provide the doctor with easily quantifiable scores. Perhaps most importantly, they can be made available continuously at the bedside (**Figure 1**).

Unfortunately, there is not one single standard monitor at this moment to accurately estimate what occurs in the brain of a coma patient. Therefore, in this chapter, we shall start with a brief exposition on coma physiopathology, insisting on burst suppression (BS) state, and we shall continue with the characteristics of the main coma states we might encounter in the intensive care unit (ICU). We will continue with the devices used to monitor anesthesia depth, which are used to monitor coma depth as well. These devices are based on EEG signal analysis. The main drawback of EEG signal analysis is noise: how shall we define and remove noise on an EEG?

A definitive answer is difficult to find, that is why "noise-resistant" mathematical algorithms have been developed. Thus, this chapter focuses on the mathematical algorithms used to interpret EEG signal, as it is important to know the basis of parameters and scores we receive from the devices we use. In the end, we describe new theories that might be standardized to evaluate coma state—such as cortical connectivity and reactivity.

2. Coma state

2.1. Coma—definition and theories

Coma is defined as a state of unconsciousness and lack of response to noxious stimuli. The physiopathology of consciousness and coma state is not entirely understood. It is not clear if a "coma center" exists or if the diverse pathological states that induce coma do so through different mechanisms. From this perspective, coma is similar to the anesthetic state, which is caused by several pharmacological agents, with different chemical structures. It is also unclear if a common center, on which all anesthetics act, exists. Based on histology and physiology, Sir Francis Crick postulated that the claustrum has a central role in maintaining consciousness (as it is connected with nearly all cerebral structures), like the conductor of an orchestra [1]. Recent studies have shown that during isoflurane anesthesia on the rat, functional connectivity of the claustrum with medial prefrontal cortex and mediodorsal thalamus decreased [2]. As for coma state, there are no definitive studies proving the role of the claustrum in its physiopathology.

Regarding EEG activity, comas are different. The same coma state, defined by a lack of consciousness and of response to external pain stimuli may exhibit different EEG aspects. Thus, there are comas with prevalent alpha waves (alpha comas), beta waves (beta comas), theta waves (theta comas) or delta waves (delta comas). A common characteristic of these coma states is that if they are secondary to intoxication or metabolic encephalopathies, they have a positive prognosis, regardless of the EEG pattern, with response to external pain stimuli. If there are secondary to brain stem lesions or hypoxic ischemic encephalopathies and lacking response to external pain stimuli, comas bring a negative prognosis [3].

Comas secondary to TBI are caused by diffuse axonal injury (DAI) and by hemorrhages that compress the brain stem. Diffuse axonal injury occurs due to rapid (rotational) acceleration, which causes lacerations in the neuronal cytoskeleton and therefore block neuronal transport [4]. Hameroff and Penrose support the hypothesis that conscious processes are based in the microtubules of the neuronal cytoskeleton [5, 6]. Furthermore, it is known that volatile anesthetics interfere with the function of these microtubules. Nevertheless, if this theory proves true—that consciousness is based on and influenced by neuronal cytoskeleton microtubules— that might explain loss of consciousness secondary to diffuse axon injury.

Another etiology of coma is nonconvulsive status, defined as prolonged seizures there are not clinically manifested and associate altered mental status [7], secondary to TBI (8–16%), to stroke—HAS (3–31%) and craniotomy [8]. The mechanism of loss of consciousness during epilepsy is not entirely understood. Blumenfeld Hal et al. affirm that a common mechanism exists—a cortico-subcortical network dysfunction. Therefore, a decrease in cerebral blood flow (CBF) was noticed in frontoparietal association areas and the anterior and posterior interhemispheric regions with (CBF) increases in bilateral midline subcortical structures [9].

Besides, a loss of connectivity between medial and lateral frontoparietal association areas and upper brainstem/medial diencephalon was observed [10]. They state that these cortico-subcortical connectivity malfunctions (occurring in generalized tonic-clonic seizures, complex partial seizures and temporal lobe seizures) are caused either by indirect inhibition or by convulsions initiated in these structures.

2.2. Burst suppression (BS) state

Burst suppression is a cortical electrical activity defined by the existence of high-amplitude and variable frequency waves discharge, followed by a period of electrical activity suppression. BS is an intermediate state between slow waves EEG pattern and an isoelectric line. This BS pattern is present in several conditions, such as Ohtahara syndrome, TBI, hypoglycemia, hypoxia, hypothermia and anesthesia [11]. As for anesthesia bursts, they have a wave morphology specific to each anesthetic compound, and a different duration as well. In addition, the length of the burst decreases as the anesthesia depth increases [12]. Not only is the burst length variable, but so is its structure, according to its length. Thus, we have noticed [13] that for isoflurane anesthesia in rat, 4-seconds bursts and 1-second bursts have different aspects

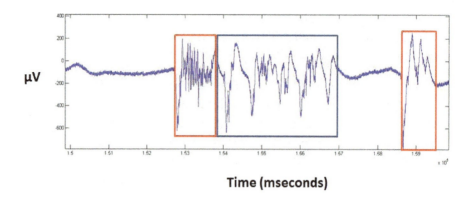

Figure 2. Burst aspects according to its length (local-field potential—LFP—recording). The first burst lasts almost 4 seconds and presents high-frequency waves at the beginning followed by slow waves. The second burst is short (almost 1 second) and presents slow waves.

(**Figure 2**). Long bursts start with high-frequency high-amplitude waves, followed by low-frequency high-amplitude waves, while short bursts present low-frequency high-amplitude waves as it is seen on power spectral density graphics (**Figure 3**).

Even though a BS presenting coma state is considered deep, BS is deemed a state of hyper-excitability, as bursts can be evoked by subliminal stimuli [14] and BS electrical activity is correlated with cerebral blood flow changes as well [15].

The mechanism supporting this phenomenon remains incompletely explained. We have two theories attempting an explanation at the moment. The metabolic theory of Emery Brown [11]

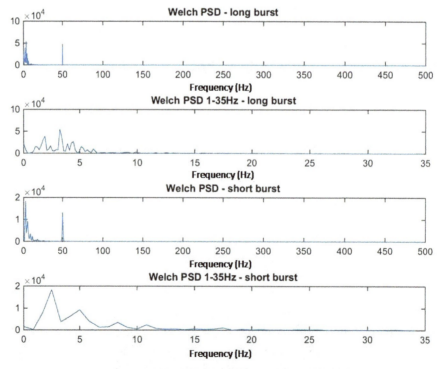

Figure 3. Power spectral density during the long burst versus the short burst. Two peaks of frequencies can be observed in the long burst.

is based on the fact that BS states correlate with low metabolism states (with low metabolic rate), such as hypothermia, anesthesia and hypoglycemia. The link between the electrical and the metabolic activity is the KATP channels, so during the burst, ATP concentration decreased which induces an increase in the conductance of KATP and thus a neuronal membrane hyperpolarization occurs (flat-line EEG). The theory of Amzica [16] states that BS activity is modulated by extracellular calcium concentration variations, thus the depletion of the extracellular cortical calcium during the burst is responsible for the EEG silence (flat line) after that. The basis of this phenomenon is unclear as well. It is regarded that bursts are caused by internal input, modulated by neural networks. On the other hand, the cortex has been proven to exhibit BS activity, without the intervention of subcortical structures [17].

In the clinical practice, finding BS patterns in coma patients presents a negative prognostic value, if the BS ratio (BSR = suppression time/epoch duration * 100) is over 20–23% [18].

3. EEG monitoring and interpretation

3.1. Continuous EEG monitoring

Continuous EEG monitoring is the most used and, perhaps, the most efficient method of evaluating coma patients in the ICU. The advantage is the electrode placing: it is noninvasive (or minimally invasive), can be easily applied on the scalp of the patient and requires a minimal qualification of the ICU staff. Most EEG recording devices include software for mathematically processing the signal, and generating scores or frequencies.

The acquisition system 10–20, that is classically used, provides an overview of the main cortical areas. Placing the electrodes and fastening them with a specialized helmet may facilitate CT or MRI transportation, in order to obtain a complex imagistic and electroencephalographic representation. Standard EEG monitoring provides information on the onset of epileptic seizures, is useful in detecting nonconvulsive status and in detecting early and late ischemia, secondary to subarachnoid hemorrhage. Furthermore, it provides useful information (based on prevailing EEG patterns and reactivity) for the prognostic of the coma patient [19].

The following chapter will describe the main mathematical algorithms that are used in analyzing EEG signal, as well as the devices used for monitoring coma and anesthesia depth.

3.2. EEG signal analysis

3.2.1. Spectral analysis

Spectral analysis of EEG signal is based on the fast Fourier transformation (FFT), which decomposes the signal according to the mean amplitude of each frequency in the signal. By applying second-order FFT, the result is the spectral power graphic, which decomposes the signal based on amplitude squared/frequency (microvolts^2/Hz). Analyzing this graphic provides very important parameters to estimate the depth of sedation/anesthesia.

Median frequency (MEF) represents the value of frequency whose perpendicular meets Ox in the point that splits equally the area under the spectral power graphic.

Spectral edge frequency (SEF) is the value of frequency from which we can draw a perpendicular to Ox that leaves 90 or 95% of the spectral power function under graphic area to the left [20] (**Figure 4**).

If the patient is anesthetized, the values of these parameters will decrease proportionally with the degree of sedation (they will shift to the left), because during sedation, the high-frequency fast waves EEG activity ceases [21]. Surgical anesthesia is performed at the moment the EEG shows mostly theta waves.

3.2.2. EEG signal entropy

Entropy represents the degree of disorder in a system. Ludwig Boltzmann defines entropy as the logarithmic function of the number of microstates corresponding to a macrostate. In 1949, Claude Shanon defines information entropy as being:

$$S = \sum_{i=1}^{n} P(x) \log P(x) \tag{1}$$

where S = entropy,

P = apparition probability,

log = binary logarithm.

As EEG is a signal composed of several types of waves, with a disorderly aspect, the more disorderly (more types of waves), the higher the entropy. An isoelectric EEG signal has a null entropy. This type of entropy, applied to EEG signals, was used to monitor anesthetic depth during desflurane anesthesia [22]. The Datex-Ohmeda company (now acquired by GE) developed a device that analyzes EEG signal entropy and displays it as a score.

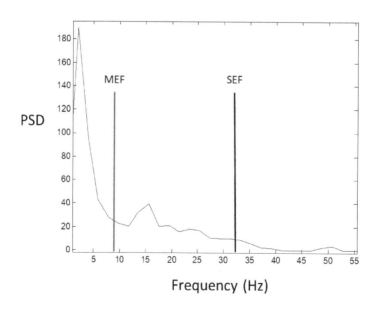

Figure 4. EEG power spectrum density (PSD). In this figure, median frequency (MEF) and spectral edge frequency (SEF) are displayed on the PSD graph.

The EEG signal entropy calculation is based on the following algorithm:

$$SN[f1, f2] = \frac{S[f1, f2]}{\log(N[f1, f2])} \quad (2)$$

where [f1, f2] = frequencies between which the EEG signal is analyzed,

N[f1, f2] = number of frequencies between f1 and f2.

The EEG signal is acquired at a frequency of 400 Hz, and to analyze it, several epochs (windows) are used, between 0.92 and 60.16 seconds, in order to cover all EEG signal frequencies. The shortest epoch is used to analyze frequencies between 32 and 47 Hz, and the 60.16 epoch to analyze frequencies under 2 Hz. The device provides two entropy indices: state entropy (SE) and response entropy (RE). SE analyzes EEG in the frequency domain 0.8–32 Hz, while RE in the 0.8–47 Hz frequency domain. The difference between RE and SE is given by the EMG activity: it is assumed that an increase of entropy in the 32–47 Hz domain corresponds to an increase of frontal electromyographic activity, and this difference shows indirectly the quality of intraoperative analgesia). SE is between 0 and 91, and RE is between 0 and 100.

During anesthesia, the values displayed by the entropy monitor must be in the range of 40–60 in order to prevent waking up during the intervention [23–25].

3.2.3. Bispectral index

The Aspect Medical company was the first to market a monitor for anesthesia depth, in 1994 [26]. It is based on the bispectral analysis of EEG signal [27]. The monitor analyzes the EEG recorded by prefrontal electrodes, based on an algorithm, undisclosed entirely up until today [28]. This algorithm calculates a score between 0 (isoelectric line) and 100 (patient awake). This algorithm was validated by correlating the clinical sedation score, lack of response to pain stimulation and EEG parameters for approximately 1500 patients (cumulating approximately 5000 hours of recordings). BIS monitoring evaluates well the degree of sedation/hypnosis of anesthesia, and not directly the anesthetic depth. It was validated for all volatile and intravenous anesthetic, except ketamine. As this generates thalamocortical dissociation, the EEG is similar to that of an awake patient. During sevoflurane anesthesia, ketamine may increase the BIS score, though anesthesia deepens [29]. In the case of propofol anesthesia, analgesic dose of ketamine does not influence the bispectral index [30–32]. Though xenon has a similar mechanism to ketamine and was not used in the validation process of the BIS monitor, it modifies the EEG similarly to propofol [33]. As for correlating the BIS score, older studies have stated that BIS under 50 does not ensure hypnosis [34]. A more recent study reveals that xenon anesthesia depth clinical signs correlate well with BIS score values [35].

The algorithm used incorporates spectral analysis, bispectral analysis and burst-suppression activity analysis (BS). Spectral analysis, described above, decomposes the signal based on the amplitude of each frequency, analyzing data individually and ignoring the relationship with other constituents. In the human brain, there are several EEG signal generators. While the patient is awake, the EEG signal is produced by the independently emitted activity of several generators, only slightly synchronized. As the patient falls asleep or is anesthetized, the number of active generators decreases and they become more synchronized. Bispectral analysis quantifies the phase-phase coupling between these EEG signal generators.

BIS components are *beta ratio* and *SyncFastSlow*. Beta ratio is the logarithm of the ratio of two frequency components of the spectral power (30–47 Hz and 11–20 Hz), while *SyncFastSlow* is the logarithm of the bispectral ratio of 0.5–47 Hz and 40–47 Hz [36].

$$BetaRatio = \log\left(\frac{P\,30-47}{P\,11-20}\right) \quad (3)$$

$$SyncFastFlow = \log\left(\frac{B\,0.5-47}{B\,40-47}\right) \quad (4)$$

BIS monitors display several parameters, such as the BIS score value (between 0 and 100), which should be maintained during anesthesia between 40 and 60 to prevent waking up, signal quality index, suppression ratio for a 60 seconds epoch (SR), the minute burst count (BC), frontal electromyographic activity (EMG)—which results from analyzing the EEG signal in the 70–110 Hz frequency interval (assumed to be produced by spontaneous frontal muscles activity) and is between 30 and 55 dB [37].

BIS monitoring can be used in the intensive care wards as well, to monitor patient sedation [38]: in traumatic brain injury, a value under 60 correlates with a negative prognosis [39]. BIS monitoring may also be used to detect cerebral vasospasm in critical patients [40]; it has been proven that it correlates well with the consciousness level of the ICU patients, it aids in adjusting sedative dosage, it has a prognostic value and it is useful in monitoring induced coma for a status epilepticus [41–44].

EMG activity is not greatly influenced by the degree of curare neuromotor block, but the pain stimulus EMG variation during anesthesia depends on the degree of neuromuscular block [45].

3.2.3.1. BIS monitoring limitations

BIS analysis of EEG signal provides information only on the sedation during anesthesia, and not on global anesthetic depth. The BIS score does not accurately predict when the patient will regain consciousness. Recent studies have shown that both loss of consciousness and waking up from anesthesia correlate with gamma cortical activity, as losing consciousness is caused by gamma rhythm cessation [46, 47]. BIS monitors cannot gather gamma rhythm EEG signal, as it can only be optimally recorded through dura mater electrodes.

BIS monitors pick up EEG signal in the prefrontal area, where spontaneous electromyographic activity interferes with gamma rhythm frequency. The BIS score cannot predict pain stimuli hemodynamic reactivity during anesthesia and is influenced by the type of anesthetic used—volatile anesthesia, for the same anesthetic potency, differently alter EEG activity. Furthermore, it is not influenced by cerebral perfusion and hypoglycemia [48].

3.2.4. Narcotrend monitoring

This monitor was marketed in 2000 by the Monitor Technik company. The EEG signal is picked up by three electrodes in the frontal area. It is then filtered and noise is removed. EEG is analyzed in the 0.5–47 Hz frequency domain. The algorithm includes the relative power of alpha, beta, theta and delta frequencies, median frequency, spectral edge frequency and spectral entropy. This monitor displays values between 0 and 100. The depth of anesthesia is divided into five stages [49]. The values provided by this monitor are well correlated with the ones provided by BIS monitoring [50]. The Narcotrend monitor has been proven useful in the postoperative care of the patients who underwent propofol sedation during cardiac surgery [51].

3.2.5. Consciousness index

The monitor for the consciousness index is a wireless, portable monitor as well, with a 10-meters range. It is produced by Morpheus Medical. It provides a score with values between 0 and 100, and, similar to the BIS monitoring during anesthesia, the value of the consciousness index must be maintained between 40 and 60 to prevent waking up during anesthesia. This monitor analyzes EEG, using symbolic dynamic analysis. As EEG is a variation of potential through time, it can be seen as a dynamic system, in which every moment has a state that can be defined through a real number. The dynamic symbol method analyzes a dynamic system as being composed of a discrete sequence of abstract symbols that each correspond to a system state [52].

This monitor was compared with BIS monitoring and similar results were found [53].

There is one other consciousness index that uses Lempel-Ziv complexity analysis. This method was established in 2013 by a team of researchers led by Adenauer Casali and Olivia Gosseries. This index was studied during midazolam sedation and propofol-xenon anesthesia, on a limited number of subjects. It is based on evaluating cortical reactivity and intercortical connectivity, using high-density EEG and transcranial magnetic stimulation on several cortical areas: superior occipital gyrus, superior medial frontal gyrus, superior parietal gyrus and premotor rostral cortex. EEG signals were analyzed using the Lempel-Ziv complexity algorithm, which approximates the amount of nonredundant information in a binary system, thus estimating the minimal amount of patterns required to describe a signal. The less EEG signal nonredundant information there is, the less complex the signal and deep the anesthesia is [54].

3.2.6. Approximate entropy

Entropy is the degree of disorder in a system, thus an extensive measurement of chaos. At the beginning of the twentieth century, the mathematicians Andrey Kolmogorov and Henri Poincare further developed the mathematical analysis of chaos. In 1991, Steven Pincus introduced the notion of approximate entropy. Approximate entropy measures the complexity of a system. As it is little influenced by noise, it has an advantage in the analysis of systems exposed to a strong source of noise. Mathematically, approximate entropy quantifies how constant the distance between two vectors in a series is [55].

The following formula is used to calculate approximate entropy:

$$\text{ApEn}(Sn, m, r) = \ln\left(\frac{C_m(r)}{C_{m+1}(r)}\right) \tag{5}$$

where m = length of the pattern,

Cm(r) = prevalence of repetitive patterns, with the length m.

Applied to time series, approximate entropy is a measurement of series predictability. As we know, electroencephalographic signal is a time variation of scalp-recorded potential. Thus, electroencephalographic signal may be described as a time series. Calculating approximate entropy, there results an estimation of EEG signal predictability, and, inherently, an estimation of the signal complexity. The more awake the patient is, the higher values the approximate entropy will have, as the EEG is more complex and less predictable. During deep sedation, EEG complexity lowers and thus will be more predictable, with a lower approximate entropy value.

Approximate value is used to estimate anesthesia depth and correlates well with BIS and SEF indices, during propofol-remifentanil anesthesia [56].

3.2.7. Permutation entropy

Permutation entropy is another method of estimating the chaos, which analyzes the probability of appearance of a motive of amplitude over a certain amount of time. The more motifs there are, the more complex the signal is, therefore the more awake the patient is. When the probability of appearance of all motifs is equal, permutation entropy equals 1. The calculation algorithm for the permutation entropy was published in 2002 by Bandt, and in 2008, Jordan et al. use this algorithm to study electroencephalograms [57, 58].

$$\text{PE} = -\frac{\sum P_i \times \ln P_i}{\ln N} \tag{6}$$

where P = probability of appearance of a motif,

N = number of motifs.

An important parameter is the signal acquisition frequency, the algorithm being designed for a frequency of 100 or 128 Hz.

In 2008, Olofsen et al. studied EEG by using permutation entropy during propofol anesthesia and described six types of motifs: peaks, slopes and grooves [59].

Using permutation entropy, the transition between loss of consciousness and consciousness can be detected by analyzing 2-seconds EEG recordings [60].

3.2.8. EEG fractality

Fractal analysis of the EEG signal implies measuring the degree of self-similarity of the signal. EEG fractal analysis was used to study sleep, anesthesia or convulsions [61–63].

Another analysis parameter for complexity, similar with fractal analysis, is detrended fluctuation analysis (DFA). It is an analysis method for signal self-similarity and was used to evaluate EEG and was suggested as a possible quantification parameter of anesthesia depth [64].

3.2.9. Auditory evoked potentials

Changes in the latency and amplitude of auditory evoked potentials of middle latency (early cortical), that appear 20–80 ms after auditory stimulation, can be correlated with anesthetic depth [65–67].

The auditory evoked potential index (AAI) is an algorithm integrating amplitude variations of several consecutive potentials and generating a numerical outcome, between 0 and 99, similar to the bispectral index [68]. Patients lose consciousness under 40, and surgical anesthesia appears under 20. AAI values are well correlated with BIS values [69]. In the ICU, middle latency evoked potentials have a positive prognostic value in the patients who required craniotomy for TBI, and there has been noticed a strong correlation between pupillary responses, intracranial pressure and auditory evoked potentials in patients with supratentorial mass lesions [70, 71].

4. Near-infrared spectroscopy (NIRS)

Jobsis first noticed in 1977 [72] that tissues are transparent for a wavelength of light of 700–950 nm. Based on this, the concentration of oxyhemoglobin, deoxyhemoglobin and cytochrome C oxidase can be measured (only the first two are used in clinical practice).

Starting from the oxyHb and deoxyHb concentrations, one can estimate regional saturation of oxygen (rSO_2) in a tissue. Furthermore, the regional changes of blood flow can be assessed, by evaluating the changes of total hemoglobin (HbT). Monitors for cerebral oxygenation, that are based on the NIRS technology, use a sensor placed above the tissue, whose oxygenation is to be measured. The sensor is made of emitting and detecting diodes, placed within 4–8 cm of each other. Detecting diodes will detect the infrared light reflected by the tissue. In the case of cerebral tissue, the infrared light can penetrate up to a depth of 0.6–1 centimeters [73]. Thus, cerebral oxygenation through this method is underestimated, compared with jugular vein saturation ($SjVO_2$) [74]. Among the benefits of this method are the noninvasive character and the ease of use at the bedside.

In the case of the brain, rSO_2 values are closer to the venous saturation than to arterial saturation because 70% of cerebral blood is in the veins and capillaries, and thus, normal cerebral rSO_2 values are between 60 and 80%. Using NIRS in the current clinical practice began in the 1980s, with the first studies on monitoring cerebral function in the adult and neonate. More recent studies are focused upon evaluating prehospital coma gravity. For example, Peters et al. [75] observed in a study including 25 patients that NIRS has a sensitivity of 93.3% and a specificity of 78.6% over CT scans in detecting intracranial hematoma.

Additionally, NIRS values have prognostic value in TBI patients. The values of rSO_2 at hospital admission were 74.7 ± 1.5% in the case of surviving patients and 61.9 ± 19.4%

in nonsurvivors [76]; therefore, rSO_2 under 60% are associated with increased mortality. In the case of resuscitated SCR patients, rSO_2 in the first 24 hours was 68.2% for survivors and 62.9% for nonsurvivors [77]. As for blood flow variation monitoring, it was noticed that the cerebral oximetry index (Cox), determined through NIRS, is a good substitute of the mean velocity index (Mx)—determined through transcranial Doppler echography (TCD) [78]. NIRS is also useful in detecting vasospasm in subarachnoid hemorrhage (SAH) patients as well [79].

5. Cortical connectivity and coma

During coma states as during the anesthesia, there is a decrease in connectivity ("communication") between different cortical regions, or between cortical and subcortical regions, caused by a reduction of cerebral activity. The basis of cortical connectivity is made of structural links, such as synapses and neural fibers.

In clinical practice, the evaluation of connectivity is performed by analyzing the coherence/correlation between biological signals (EEG, ECoG and local-field potentials) from different regions of the brain.

Functional connectivity is based on biological signals analysis, which can be described as time series (such as the EEG) and can quantify cortical connectivity using statistical analysis (correlation) of the EEG signals from different cortical areas. The better the EEG signals are correlated (estimated by the correlation coefficient, XAppEn, mscohere), the more they are alike; therefore, there is a good connectivity between the cortical areas. Importantly, good statistical correlation of biological signals does not necessarily involve causality, and does not point out the direction the information moves [80]. Unlike structural connectivity, functional connectivity is time-dependent [81].

Effective connectivity may be regarded as a unit of structural and functional connectivity. It is the latest instrument trying to establish causal relations between neural network components [81]. Effective connectivity is calculated using complex mathematical algorithms (such as Granger causality or transfer entropy), applied to time series.

The state of consciousness, according to Buzsaki (2007), is the consequence of the functional transformation of information contained by a neural network. Both posterior parietal and prefrontal association areas and frontoparietal network information integration were considered involved in the generation and maintenance of the state of consciousness [82, 83]. During sleep, which is a reversible modification of consciousness as well, there is a modification of cortical connectivity; therefore, during NREM sleep, it lowers and during REM sleep, it increases [84].

Cortical connectivity changes during anesthesia were first observed in lab animals, and then in humans. Thus, in 2005, the cortical connectivity changes, especially in the prefrontal cortex, during sevoflurane anesthesia of different concentrations, were described. Bouveroux et al. described the effects of propofol on cortical connectivity: during propofol anesthesia, corticocortical and thalamocortical connectivity decreases in frontal-parietal networks, while it is maintained in the visual and auditory cortex [85]. Mhuircheartaigh et al. regard the lack of response to auditory and pain stimuli during propofol anesthesia as a consequence of putamen-cortex connectivity decreases, while thalamocortical connectivity remains unchanged [86]. Ferrarelli et al. notice as well the frontal intracortical connectivity decreases, during transcranial magnetic stimulation, under midazolam sedation [87]. Cortical connectivity is disrupted in several pathological states, such as brain trauma, vegetative state and memory or attention loss.

During mild brain trauma, there have been described frontal and occipital cortical connectivity changes, a decrease of intercortical connectivity over longer distances and an increase of cortical connectivity over shorter distances [88]. The vegetative state is defined as the abolishing of consciousness, while excitatory external factors are present. While in vegetative state, there is a decrease of cortical connectivity in several areas: prefrontal and premotor cortex, temporal-parietal association areas and posterior cingulate cortex. Furthermore, there is an altered connectivity between prefrontal and premotor cortical areas and posterior cingulate cortex [89]. Subcortical cerebrovascular accidents alter cortical connectivity between the two hemispheres: between supplementary motor areas and between ipsilateral supplementary motor area and lateral premotor area. These neural connectivity modifications, both under physiological and under pathological conditions, make cortical connectivity, if not the most sensitive, among the most sensitive parameters of nervous function.

5.1. Evaluating cortical connectivity

5.1.1. Mathematical algorithms to estimate cortical connectivity

Functional cortical connectivity may be estimated by calculating the correlation coefficient between signals of different regions, the covariance or the coherence of two or several signals. The disadvantage of these algorithms is the inability to determine the direction of data exchange between cortical and subcortical areas.

Effective cortical connectivity is estimated with the direct transfer function (DTF), based on Granger causality. Named after Clive Granger, econometrician awarded the Nobel Memorial Prize in Economic Sciences in 2003, the Granger linear systems causality states that for two time series (such as two EEG channels) with a unidirectional data exchange from the Y series to the X series, the modifications from the Y series will be found after a certain amount of time in the X series, or that analyzing Y series data can better predict X series modifications. By evaluating effective connectivity through DTF, we may analyze several time series/ EEG channels. This algorithm was developed by Polish mathematicians Kaminski and Blinowska in 1991 [90].

BSMART is a cortical connectivity analysis software package that can run on the MATLAB program.

Cortical connectivity can also be evaluated through imagistic methods (such as MRI) or electrophysiological methods (EEG).

High-density electroencephalography (64–256 electrodes) can provide information on intercortical connectivity, and is based on EEG signal analysis of different cortical regions. It has the advantage of being usable bedside, and data analysis can be performed more quickly than in the case of imagistic methods [91, 92].

6. Cortical reactivity and coma state

Evaluating cortical reactivity in coma patients seems to be a useful prognostic tool. In 1995, Gütling noticed that cortical reactivity to external stimuli at 48 and 72 hours correlates well with the neurological outcome at 1.5 years after the incident, in the case of severe head injury [93]. More recent studies, performed by Logi and Rossetti, have shown that the presence of EEG reactivity in coma caused by a traumatic brain injury, a cerebrovascular disease or postanoxic coma after a cardiac arrest associates a good outcome [94, 95]. Although these studies on using cortical reactivity in the evaluation of coma patients prognostic were published in the 1990s, there is no standardization in this matter, neither of evoked potential type, nor of reactivity-evaluating algorithm one should use.

Particularly useful is the BS state, usually correlated with a negative prognostic. Although regarded as a deep coma state, applying visual, auditory or somatosensory stimuli under the BS state gives rise to evoked bursts under isoflurane anesthesia, as proven by Hartikainen [96]. During burst suppression states, cortical reactivity seems to rise proportionally with the suppression, with maximal cortical reactivity at a BS ratio of 40–80%. Additional studies are required to validate a parameter for the cortical reactivity of coma patients.

Author details

Bogdan Pavel[1,2]*

*Address all correspondence to: pavelbogdan2009@gmail.com

1 Division of Physiology and Neurosciences, University of Medicine and Pharmacy "Carol Davila", Bucharest, Romania

2 Emergency Hospital Plastic Surgery and Burns, Bucharest, Romania

References

[1] Crick FC, Koch C. What is the function of the claustrum? Philosophical Transactions of the Royal Society of London. Series B, Biological Sciences. 2005;**360**(1458):1271-1279

[2] Smith JB, Liang Z, Watson GDR, Alloway KD, Zhang N. Interhemispheric resting-state functional connectivity of the claustrum in the awake and anesthetized states. Brain Structure & Function. 2017;**222**(5):2041-2058

[3] Sutter R, Kaplan PW. Electroencephalographic patterns in coma: When things slow down. Epileptologie. 2012;**29**:201-209

[4] Johnson VE, Stewart W, Smith DH. Axonal pathology in traumatic brain injury. Experimental Neurology. 2013;**246**:35-43

[5] Hameroff S, Penrose R. Consciousness in the universe: A review of the 'Orch OR' theory. Physics of Life Reviews. 2014;**11**(1):39-78

[6] Penrose R. Shadows of the Mind: An Approach to the Missing Science of Consciousness. Oxford: Oxford University Press; 1994

[7] Chang AK, Shinnar S. Nonconvulsive status epilepticus. Emergency Medicine Clinics of North America. 2011;**29**(1):65-72

[8] Kubota Y, Nakamoto H, Kawamata T. Nonconvulsive status epilepticus in the neurosurgical setting. Neurologia Medico-Chirurgica (Tokyo). 2016;**56**(10):626-631

[9] Yu L, Blumenfeld H. Theories of impaired consciousness in epilepsy. Annals of the New York Academy of Sciences. 2009;**1157**:48-60

[10] Blumenfeld H. Impaired consciousness in epilepsy. Lancet Neurology. 2012;**11**(9):814-826

[11] Ching S, Purdon PL, Vijayan S, Kopell NJ, Brown EN. A neurophysiological-metabolic model for burst suppression. Proceedings of the National Academy of Sciences of the United States of America. 2012;**109**(8):3095-3100

[12] Akrawi WP, Drummond JC, Kalkman CJ, Patel PM. A comparison of the electrophysiologic characteristics of EEG burst-suppression as produced by isoflurane, thiopental, etomidate, and propofol. Journal of Neurosurgical Anesthesiology. 1996;**8**(1):40-46

[13] Pavel B, Acatrinei CA, Menardy F, Zahiu CMD, Popa D, Zagrean AM, Zagrean L. Changes of cortical connectivity during deep anaesthesia. Romanian Journal of Anaesthesia and Intensive Care. 2015;**22**(2):83-88

[14] Kroeger D, Amzica F. Hypersensitivity of the anesthesia-induced comatose brain. The Journal of Neuroscience. 2007;**27**(39):10597-10607

[15] Liu X, Zhu XH, Zhang Y, Chen W. Neural origin of spontaneous hemodynamic fluctuations in rats under burst-suppression anesthesia condition. Cerebral Cortex. 2011;**21**(2):374-384

[16] Amzica F. Basic physiology of burst-suppression. Epilepsia. 2009;**50**(Suppl 12):38-39

[17] Topolnik L, Steriade M, Timofeev I. Partial cortical deafferentation promotes development of paroxysmal activity. Cerebral Cortex. 2003;**13**(8):883-893

[18] Theilen HJ, Ragaller M, Tschö U, May SA, Schackert G, Albrecht MD. Electroencephalogram silence ratio for early outcome prognosis in severe head trauma. Critical Care Medicine. 2000;**28**(10):3522-3529

[19] Caricato A, Melchionda I, Antonelli M. Continuous electroencephalography monitoring in adults in the intensive care unit. Critical Care. 2018;**22**(1):75

[20] Tonner PH, Bein B. Classic electroencephalographic parameters: Median frequency, spectral edge frequency etc. Best Practice & Research. Clinical Anaesthesiology. 2006;**20**(1):147-159

[21] Martín-Cancho MF, Lima JR, Luis L, Crisóstomo V, López MA, Ezquerra LJ, Carrasco-Jiménez MS, Usón-Gargallo J. Bispectral index, spectral edge frequency 95% and median frequency recorded at varying desflurane concentrations in pigs. Research in Veterinary Science. 2006;**81**(3):373-381

[22] Bruhn J, Lehmann LE, Röpcke H, Bouillon TW, Hoeft A. Shannon entropy applied to the measurement of the electroencephalographic effects of desflurane. Anesthesiology. 2001;**95**(1):30-35

[23] Viertiö-Oja H, Maja V, Särkelä M, Talja P, Tenkanen N, Tolvanen-Laakso H, Paloheimo M, Vakkuri A, Yli-Hankala A, Meriläinen P. Description of the entropy algorithm as applied in the Datex-Ohmeda S/5 entropy module. Acta Anaesthesiologica Scandinavica. 2004;**48**(2):154-161

[24] Vakkuri A, Yli-Hankala A, Sandin R, Mustola S, Høymork S, Nyblom S, Talja P, Sampson T, van Gils M, Viertiö-Oja H. Spectral entropy monitoring is associated with reduced propofol use and faster emergence in propofol-nitrous oxide-alfentanil anesthesia. Anesthesiology. 2005;**103**(2):274-279

[25] Vakkuri A, Yli-Hankala A, Talja P, Mustola S, Tolvanen-Laakso H, Sampson T, Viertiö-Oja H. Time-frequency balanced spectral entropy as a measure of anesthetic drug effect in central nervous system during sevoflurane, propofol, and thiopental anesthesia. Acta Anaesthesiologica Scandinavica. 2004;**48**(2):145-153

[26] Sigl JC, Chamoun NG. An introduction to bispectral analysis for the electroencephalogram. Journal of Clinical Monitoring. 1994;**10**(6):392-404

[27] Abarbanel H, Davis R, MacDonald GJ, Munk W. Bispectra. Defense Technical Information Center, Document ADA150870; 1984

[28] Bruhn J, Bouillon TW, Shafer SL. Bispectral index (BIS) and burst suppression: Revealing a part of the BIS algorithm. Journal of Clinical Monitoring and Computing. 2000;**16**(8):593-596

[29] Hans P, Dewandre PY, Brichant JF, Bonhomme V. Comparative effects of ketamine on bispectral index and spectral entropy of the electroencephalogram under sevofluraneanaesthesia. British Journal of Anaesthesia. 2005;**94**(3):336-340

[30] Faraoni D, Salengros JC, Engelman E, Ickx B, Barvais L. Ketamine has no effect on bispectral index during stable propofol-remifentanilanaesthesia. British Journal of Anaesthesia. 2009;**102**(3):336-339

[31] Sengupta S, Ghosh S, Rudra A, Kumar P, Maitra G, Das T. Effect of ketamine on bispectral index during propofol–fentanyl anesthesia: A randomized controlled study. Middle East Journal of Anesthesiology. 2011;**21**(3):391-395

[32] Nonaka A, Makino K, Suzuki S, Ikemoto K, Furuya A, Tamaki F, Asano N. Low doses of ketamine have no effect on bispectral index during stable propofol-remifentanil anesthesia. Masui. 2012;**61**(4):364-367

[33] Laitio RM, Kaskinoro K, Särkelä MO, Kaisti KK, Salmi E, Maksimow A, Långsjö JW, Aantaa R, Kangas K, Jääskeläinen S, Scheinin H. Bispectral index, entropy, and quantitative electroencephalogram during single-agent xenon anesthesia. Anesthesiology. 2008;**108**(1):63-70

[34] Goto T, Nakata Y, Saito H, Ishiguro Y, Niimi Y, Suwa K, Morita S. Bispectral analysis of the electroencephalogram does not predict responsiveness to verbal command in patients emerging from xenon anaesthesia. British Journal of Anaesthesia. 2000;**85**(3):359-363

[35] Fahlenkamp AV, Krebber F, Rex S, Grottke O, Fries M, Rossaint R, Coburn M. Bispectral index monitoring during balanced xenon or sevoflurane anaesthesia in elderly patients. European Journal of Anaesthesiology. 2010;**27**(10):906-911

[36] Antognini JF, Carstens E, Raines DE. Neural Mechanism of Anesthesia. NJ, USA: Humana Press; 2002

[37] Nunes RR, Chaves IM, de Alencar JC, Franco SB, de Oliveira YG, de Menezes DG. Bispectral index and other processed parameters of electroencephalogram: an update. Rev Bras Anestesiol. Jan-Feb, 2012;**62**(1):105-117

[38] Zhao D, Xu Y, He W, Li T, He Y. A comparison of bispectral index and sedation agitation scale in guiding sedation therapy: A randomized controlled study in patients undergoing short term mechanical ventilation. Zhongguo Wei Zhong Bing Ji Jiu Yi Xue. 2011;**23**(4):220-223

[39] Li HL, Miao WL, Ren HX, Lin HY, Wang HP. The value of bispectral index in the unconscious patients with acute brain injury due to different pathogenic factors. Zhonghua Wei Zhong Bing Ji Jiu Yi Xue. 2013;**25**(3):174-176

[40] Brallier JW, Deiner SG. Use of the bilateral BIS monitor as an indicator of cerebral vasospasm in ICU patients. Middle East Journal of Anesthesiology. 2013;**22**(2):161-164. PubMed PMID: 24180164

[41] Mondello E, Siliotti R, Noto G, Cuzzocrea E, Scollo G, Trimarchi G, Venuti FS. Bispectral index in ICU: Correlation with Ramsay score on assessment of sedation level. Journal of Clinical Monitoring and Computing. 2002;**17**(5):271-277

[42] Mahmood S, Parchani A, El-Menyar A, Zarour A, Al-Thani H, Latifi R. Utility of bispectral index in the management of multiple trauma patients. Surgical Neurology International. 2014;**5**:141

[43] Dou L, Gao HM, Lu L, Chang WX. Bispectral index in predicting the prognosis of patients with coma in intensive care unit. World Journal of Emergency Medicine. 2014;**5**(1):53-56.

[44] Musialowicz T, Mervaala E, Kälviäinen R, Uusaro A, Ruokonen E, Parviainen I. Can BIS monitoring be used to assess the depth of propofol anesthesia in the treatment of refractory status epilepticus? Epilepsia. 2010;**51**(8):1580-1586

[45] Ekman A, Stålberg E, Sundman E, Eriksson LI, Brudin L, Sandin R. The effect of neuromuscular block and noxious stimulation on hypnosis monitoring during sevoflurane anesthesia. Anesthesia and Analgesia. 2007;**105**(3):688-695

[46] John ER, Prichep LS. The anesthetic cascade: A theory of how anesthesia suppresses consciousness. Anesthesiology. 2005;**102**:447-471

[47] Imas OA, Ropella KM, Ward BD, Wood JD, Hudetz AG. Volatile anesthetics disrupt frontal-posterior recurrent information transfer at gamma frequencies in rat. Neuroscience Letters. 2005;**387**:145-150

[48] Duarte LT, Saraiva RA. When the bispectral index (bis) can give false results. Revista Brasileira de Anestesiologia. 2009;**59**(1):99-109. Review

[49] Kreuer S, Wilhelm W. The Narcotrend monitor. Best Practice & Research. Clinical Anaesthesiology. 2006;**20**(1):111-119. Review. PubMed PMID: 16634418

[50] Schultz A, Siedenberg M, Grouven U, Kneif T, Schultz B. Comparison of narcotrend index, bispectral index, spectral and entropy parameters during induction of propofol-remifentanilanaesthesia. Journal of Clinical Monitoring and Computing. 2008;**22**(2):103-111

[51] Weber F, Steinberger M, Ritzka M, Prasser C, Bein T. Measuring depth of sedation in intensive care patients with the electroencephalographic narcotrend index. European Journal of Anaesthesiology. 2008;**25**(2):123-128

[52] Musizza B, Ribaric S. Monitoring the depth of anaesthesia. Sensors (Basel). 2010;**10**(12): 10896-10935

[53] Chakravarthy M, Holla S, Jawali V. Index of consciousness and bispectral index values are interchangeable during normotension and hypotension but not during non pulsatile flow state during cardiac surgical procedures: A prospective study. Journal of Clinical Monitoring and Computing. 2010;**24**(2):83-91

[54] Casali AG, Gosseries O, Rosanova M, Boly M, Sarasso S, Casali KR, Casarotto S, Bruno MA, Laureys S, Tononi G, Massimini M. A theoretically based index of consciousness independent of sensory processing and behavior. Science Translational Medicine. 2013;**5**(198):198ra105

[55] Pincus SM. Approximate entropy as a measure of system complexity. Proceedings of the National Academy of Sciences of the United States of America. 1991;**88**(6):2297-2301

[56] Bruhn J, Bouillon TW, Radulescu L, Hoeft A, Bertaccini E, Shafer SL. Correlation of approximate entropy, bispectral index, and spectral edge frequency 95 (SEF95) with clinical signs of "anesthetic depth" during coadministration of propofol and remifentanil. Anesthesiology. 2003;**98**(3):621-627

[57] Bandt C, Pompe B. Permutation entropy: A natural complexity measure for time series. Physical Review Letters. 2002;**88**(17):174102

[58] Jordan D, Stockmanns G, Kochs EF, Pilge S, Schneider G. Electroencephalographic order pattern analysis for the separation of consciousness and unconsciousness: An analysis of approximate entropy, permutation entropy, recurrence rate, and phase coupling of order recurrence plots. Anesthesiology. 2008;**109**(6):1014-1022

[59] Olofsen E, Sleigh JW, Dahan A. Permutation entropy of the electroencephalogram: A measure of anaesthetic drug effect. British Journal of Anaesthesia. 2008;**101**(6):810-821

[60] Kreuzer M, Kochs EF, Schneider G, Jordan D. Non-stationarity of EEG during wakefulness and anaesthesia: Advantages of EEG permutation entropy monitoring. Journal of Clinical Monitoring and Computing; 2014

[61] Yeh JR, Peng CK, Lo MT, Yeh CH, Chen SC, Wang CY, Lee PL, Kang JH. Investigating the interaction between heart rate variability and sleep EEG using nonlinear algorithms. Journal of Neuroscience Methods. 2013;**219**(2):233-239

[62] Willand M, Rudner R, Olejarczyk E, Wartak M, Marciniak R, Stasiowski M, Byrczek T, Jałowiecki P. Fractal dimension–A new EEG-based method of assessing the depth of anaesthesia. Anestezjologia Intensywna Terapia. 2008;**40**(4):217-222

[63] Wang Y, Zhou W, Yuan Q, Li X, Meng Q, Zhao X, Wang J. Comparison of ictaland interictal EEG signals using fractal features. International Journal of Neural Systems. 2013;**23**(6):1350028

[64] Jospin M, Caminal P, Jensen EW, Litvan H, Vallverdú M, Struys MM, Vereecke HE, Kaplan DT. Detrended fluctuation analysis of EEG as a measure of depth of anesthesia. IEEE Transactions on Biomedical Engineering. 2007;**54**(5):840-846

[65] Thornton C, Barrowcliffe MP, Konieczko KM, Ventham P, Doré CJ, Newton DE, Jones JG. The auditory evoked response as an indicator of awareness. British Journal of Anaesthesia. 1989;**63**(1):113-115

[66] Schwender D, Kaiser A, Klasing S, Peter K, Pöppel E. Midlatency auditory evoked potentials and explicit and implicit memory in patients undergoing cardiac surgery. Anesthesiology. 1994;**80**(3):493-501

[67] Newton DE, Thornton C, Konieczko KM, Jordan C, Webster NR, Luff NP, Frith CD, Doré CJ. Auditory evoked response and awareness: A study in volunteers at sub-MAC concentrations of isoflurane. British Journal of Anaesthesia. 1992;**69**(2):122-129

[68] Mantzaridis H, Kenny GN. Auditory evoked potential index: A quantitative measure of changes in auditory evoked potentials during general anaesthesia. Anaesthesia. 1997;**52**(11):1030-1036

[69] Schraag S, Bothner U, Gajraj R, Kenny GN, Georgieff M. The performance of electroencephalogram bispectral index and auditory evoked potential index to predict loss of consciousness during propofol infusion. Anesthesia and Analgesia. 1999;**89**(5):1311-1315

[70] Tsurukiri J, Nagata K, Hoshiai A, Oomura T, Jimbo H, Ikeda Y. Middle latency auditory-evoked potential index monitoring of cerebral function to predict functional outcome after emergency craniotomy in patients with brain damage. Scandinavian Journal of Trauma, Resuscitation and Emergency Medicine. 2015;**23**:80

[71] Krieger D, Adams HP, Schwarz S, Rieke K, Aschoff A, Hacke W. Prognostic and clinical relevance of pupillary responses, intracranial pressure monitoring, and brainstem auditory evoked potentials in comatose patients with acute supratentorial mass lesions. Critical Care Medicine. 1993;**21**(12):1944-1950

[72] Jöbsis FF. Noninvasive, infrared monitoring of cerebral and myocardial oxygen sufficiency and circulatory parameters. Science. 1977;**198**(4323):1264-1267

[73] Kleinfeld D, Mitra PP, Helmchen F, Denk W. Fluctuations and stimulus-induced changes in blood flow observed in individual capillaries in layers 2 through 4 of rat neocortex. Proceedings of the National Academy of Sciences of the United States of America. 1998;**95**(26):15741-15746

[74] Kim MB, Ward DS, Cartwright CR, Kolano J, Chlebowski S, Henson LC. Estimation of jugular venous O2 saturation from cerebral oximetry or arterial O2 saturation during isocapnic hypoxia. Journal of Clinical Monitoring and Computing. 2000;**16**(3):191-199

[75] Peters J, Van Wageningen B, Hoogerwerf N, Tan E. Near-infrared spectroscopy: A promising prehospital tool for management of traumatic brain injury. Prehospital and Disaster Medicine. 2017;**32**(4):414-418

[76] Vilkė A, Bilskienė D, Šaferis V, Gedminas M, Bieliauskaitė D, Tamašauskas A, Macas A. Predictive value of early near-infrared spectroscopy monitoring of patients with traumatic brain injury. Medicina (Kaunas, Lithuania). 2014;**50**(5):263-268

[77] Ahn A, Yang J, Inigo-Santiago L, Parnia S. A feasibility study of cerebral oximetry monitoring during the post-resuscitation period in comatose patients following cardiac arrest. Resuscitation. 2014;**85**(4):522-526

[78] Rivera-Lara L, Geocadin R, Zorrilla-Vaca A, Healy R, Radzik BR, Palmisano C, Mirski M, Ziai WC, Hogue C. Validation of near-infrared spectroscopy for monitoring cerebral autoregulation in comatose patients. Neurocritical Care. 2017;**27**(3):362-369

[79] Yokose N, Sakatani K, Murata Y, Awano T, Igarashi T, Nakamura S, Hoshino T, Katayama Y. Bedside monitoring of cerebral blood oxygenation and hemodynamics after aneurysmal subarachnoid hemorrhage by quantitative time-resolved near-infrared spectroscopy. World Neurosurgery. 2010;**73**(5):508-513

[80] Smith SM, Vidaurre D, Beckmann CF, Glasser MF, Jenkinson M, Miller KL, Nichols TE, Robinson EC, Salimi-Khorshidi G, Woolrich MW, Barch DM, Uğurbil K, Van Essen DC. Functional connectomics from resting-state fMRI. Trends in Cognitive Sciences. 2013;**17**(12):666-682

[81] Sporns O. Structure and function of complex brain networks. Dialogues in Clinical Neuroscience. 2013;**15**(3):247-262

[82] Buzsáki G. The structure of consciousness. Nature. 2007;**446**(7133):267

[83] Naghavi HR, Nyberg L. Common fronto-parietal activity in attention, memory, and consciousness: Shared demands on integration? Consciousness and Cognition. 2005;**14**(2):390-425

[84] Massimini M, Ferrarelli F, Murphy M, Huber R, Riedner B, Casarotto S, Tononi G. Cortical reactivity and effective connectivity during REM sleep in humans. Cognitive Neuroscience. 2010;**1**(3):176-183

[85] Boveroux P, Vanhaudenhuyse A, Bruno MA, Noirhomme Q, Lauwick S, Luxen A, Degueldre C, Plenevaux A, Schnakers C, Phillips C, Brichant JF, Bonhomme V, Maquet

P, Greicius MD, Laureys S, Boly M. Breakdown of within- and between-network resting state functional magnetic resonance imaging connectivity during propofol-induced loss of consciousness. Anesthesiology. 2010;**113**(5):1038-1053

[86] Mhuircheartaigh RN, Rosenorn-Lanng D, Wise R, Jbabdi S, Rogers R, Tracey I. Cortical and subcortical connectivity changes during decreasing levels of consciousness in humans: A functional magnetic resonance imaging study using propofol. The Journal of Neuroscience. 2010;**30**(27):9095-9102

[87] Ferrarelli F, Massimini M, Sarasso S, Casali A, Riedner BA, Angelini G, Tononi G, Pearce RA. Breakdown in cortical effective connectivity during midazolam-induced loss of consciousness. Proceedings of the National Academy of Sciences of the United States of America. 2010;**107**(6):2681-2686

[88] Cao C, Slobounov S. Alteration of cortical functional connectivity as a result of traumatic brain injury revealed by graph theory, ICA, and sLORETA analyses of EEG signals. IEEE Transactions on Neural Systems and Rehabilitation Engineering. 2010;**18**(1):11-19

[89] Laureys S, Goldman S, Phillips C, Van Bogaert P, Aerts J, Luxen A, Franck G, Maquet P. Impaired effective cortical connectivity in vegetative state: Preliminary investigation using PET. NeuroImage. 1999;**9**(4):377-382

[90] Kamiński MJ, Blinowska KJ. A new method of the description of the information flow in the brain structures. Biological Cybernetics. 1991;**65**(3):203-210

[91] Murphy M, Bruno MA, Riedner BA, Boveroux P, Noirhomme Q, Landsness EC, Brichant JF, Phillips C, Massimini M, Laureys S, Tononi G, Boly M. Propofol anesthesia and sleep: A high-density EEG study. Sleep. 2011;**34**(3):283-91A

[92] Astolfi L, de Vico Fallani F, Cincotti F, Mattia D, Marciani MG, Bufalari S, Salinari S, Colosimo A, Ding L, Edgar JC, Heller W, Miller GA, He B, Babiloni F. Imaging functional brain connectivity patterns from high-resolution EEG and fMRI via graph theory. Psychophysiology. 2007;**44**(6):880-893

[93] Gütling E, Gonser A, Imhof HG, Landis T. EEG reactivity in the prognosis of severe head injury. Neurology. 1995;**45**(5):915-918

[94] Logi F, Pasqualetti P, Tomaiuolo F. Predict recovery of consciousness in post-acute severe brain injury: The role of EEG reactivity. Brain Injury. 2011;**25**(10):972-979

[95] Rossetti AO, Oddo M, Logroscino G, Kaplan PW. Prognostication after cardiac arrest and hypothermia: A prospective study. Annals of Neurology. 2010;**67**(3):301-307

[96] Hartikainen KM, Rorarius M, Peräkylä JJ, Laippala PJ, Jäntti V. Cortical reactivity during isoflurane burst-suppression anesthesia. Anesthesia and Analgesia. 1995;**81**(6):1223-1228

Sepsis in Children

Selim Öncel

Abstract

Sepsis is systemic inflammatory response syndrome due to a documented or suspected infection. Causative agents of sepsis include group B streptococcus, *Escherichia coli*, and *Listeria monocytogenes* in infants younger than 2 months, and community-acquired organisms. Bacteremia may ensue in patients whose defense mechanisms have become vulnerable due to many factors. Sepsis and septic shock can be viewed as clinical pictures, which develop as consequences of proinflammatory processes/cytokines leading to a state that cannot be restrained by anti-inflammatory processes/cytokines. As yet, a cytokine, which is uniquely associated with severe sepsis and septic shock and can be used as a biomarker, has not been discovered. Sepsis is a cytokine storm, which may adversely affect almost any organ system. Whether there is an association between the severity of sepsis or septic shock and cytokine gene polymorphisms is an important field of study. Mottled skin and prolongation of capillary refill time may help the physician recognize septic shock before hypotension emerges. The management of severe sepsis and septic shock involves (1) the hemodynamic support, (2) inotropes, vasopressors, and vasodilators, (3) antimicrobial therapy, (4) transfusions, and (5) corticosteroids as indicated. Hospital mortality of pediatric sepsis is 2–10%.

Keywords: sepsis, pediatrics, cytokines, sepsis-associated encephalopathy, systemic inflammatory response syndrome, neonatal sepsis

1. Introduction

Although sepsis can affect any individual at any time during her/his lifetime, it is more apt to occur and be destructive at the extremes of life, the very old and the very young.

It is sometimes referred to as "blood poisoning" in anglophone countries and in various manners elsewhere (e.g., "microbe in blood" in Turkey). The sepsis is the body's deadly response to infection. Once sets in, sepsis can progress to septic shock and death if left untreated. One-third of people who develop sepsis die worldwide. These deaths occur more frequently in economically developing countries [1].

This chapter deals with pediatric sepsis with much greater emphasis on beyond neonatal period.

2. Definitions

Systemic inflammatory response syndrome (SIRS) is defined as two or more of the following items, one of which has to be the one marked with an asterisk (*) [2]:

1. Body core temperature of higher than 38.5°C or lower than 36°C*.

2. Except leukopenia caused by chemotherapy, a leukocyte count exceeding or lower than normal limit for age or immature leukocyte count above 10% of total leukocyte count*.

3. Abnormal heart rate:

    (a) In children 1 year of age and over

    - Average heart rate in excess of two standard deviations from the age normal in the absence of external stimuli, long-term drug use, or painful stimuli
    - Persistent elevation in heart rate in 24 h without any other explanation

    (b) In children less than 1 year of age

    - Average heart rate below 10th percentile for age in the absence of external vagal stimulus, beta-blocker, or congenital heart disease
    - Persistent depression in heart rate in half an hour without any other explanation

4. Average respiratory rate of more than two standard deviations above normal for mechanical ventilation that is being carried out for an acute process irrelevant of general anesthesia or an underlying neuromuscular disease.

Sepsis is SIRS due to a documented or suspected infection [2–5].

Organ dysfunction definitions are explained below:

1. If at least one of the following items is present despite isotonic intravenous fluid bolus (≥40 mL/kg in 1 h), this is called **cardiovascular dysfunction** [2]:

    (a) Criteria for drop in blood pressure:

- Blood pressure is below fifth percentile for age OR.
- Systolic blood pressure below two standard deviations of normal for age.

(b) Vasoactive drugs required for maintaining normal blood pressure (5 μg/kg/min dopamine or dobutamine of any dosage, epinephrine, or norepinephrine).

(c) Presence of more than two of the following items:

- Unexplained metabolic acidosis with a base deficit of more than 5 mmol/L.
- Arterial lactate concentration of more than two times the upper limit.
- Urine output of less than 0.5 mL/kg/h.
- Capillary refill time of more than 5 s.
- The difference between core and peripheral temperature of more than 3°C.

2. If at least one of the following items is present, this is called **respiratory dysfunction** [2]:

   (a) Arterial oxygen partial pressure (PaO_2)/inspired oxygen fraction (FiO_2) ratio of less than 300 in the absence of pulmonary disease or cyanotic heart disease.

   (b) Initial measurement of arterial carbon dioxide partial pressure ($PaCO_2$) above 65 Torr or 20 mmHg.

   (c) Proven requirement for maintaining the saturation at or above 92% or FiO_2 of more than 50%.

   (d) Nonelective invasive or noninvasive mechanical ventilation requirement.

3. If at least one of the following items is present, this is called **neurological dysfunction** [2]:

   (a) Glasgow Coma Score of 11 or less.

   (b) Acute change in mental status together with a drop of Glasgow Coma Score of three or more points from abnormal baseline value.

4. If at least one of the following items is present, the situation is called **hematological dysfunction** [2]:

   (a) International normalized ratio (INR) above 2.

   (b) Platelet count below 80,000/μL or has decreased 50% from the highest value recorded in the last 3 days (for chronic hematology-oncology patients).

5. **Renal dysfunction** is serum creatinine concentration of two times the upper limit for normal or more or twofold increase in baseline serum creatinine [2].

6. The presence of at least two of the following items is called **liver dysfunction** [2]:

    (a) Alanine transaminase (ALT) concentration of two times the upper limit for age.

    (b) Total bilirubin concentration of 4 mg/dL or more (not applicable for newborns).

For establishing the diagnosis of **acute respiratory distress syndrome (ARDS)**, the following criteria should be met [2]:

- PaO_2/FiO_2 ratio <200 mmHg.

- Bilateral infiltrates on chest X-ray.

- Acute onset.

- No sign of left heart failure present.

If, in addition to sepsis, there is cardiovascular organ dysfunction, ARDS, or two or more other organ dysfunctions, this situation is called **severe sepsis** [2].

3. Causative agents

Sepsis may be a consequence of infections due to bacteria, viruses, fungi, or parasites. Causative agents of sepsis include group B streptococcus, *Escherichia coli*, *Listeria monocytogenes* in infants younger than 2 months of age, and community-acquired organisms like *S. pneumoniae* and *Neisseria meningitidis* in children of 1–2 years. In a Canadian study of 6-year duration, the most common pathogens in bloodstream infections of childhood were *S. pneumoniae*, *Staphylococcus aureus*, and *E. coli* [6].

4. Pathophysiology

The site of infection, as the cause of sepsis, varies according to age. In infants, it is usually primary bacteremia. There is respiratory tract infection in nearly half of older children with sepsis [7].

Since sepsis is defined as SIRS, or in other words, pathological changes in body temperature, heart, or respiratory rates, and leukocyte count in the presence of proven or suspected infection, it would be prudent that we review the pathogeneses of the components of SIRS and infection that form sepsis and changes due to organ dysfunction in severe sepsis separately [2, 8].

4.1. Formation of infection

One of the most important clinical situations causing sepsis and septic shock is bacteremia. Bacteria must pass through the dermal or mucosal barrier in order that bacteremia takes place.

The pathogenesis of bacteremia is closely associated with the self-defense of the host and the characteristics of the bacteria. Organisms like *S. pneumoniae*, *N. meningitidis* and *Haemophilus influenzae* type b, which form a part of nasopharyngeal flora, cause bacteremia by overcoming mucosal defense systems with the aid of facilitating factors like upper respiratory infections. *N. meningitidis* is taken into the cylindrical epithelial cell with phagocytosis. After traversing the cytoplasm in the phagosome, it passes into subepithelial tissues. *H. influenzae* type b passes into subepithelial tissues by clinging to the epithelial cell and loosing the intercellular tight junctions making its way toward pharyngeal capillaries. *S. pneumoniae* attaches to specific receptors by means of which it enters the cell. The number of platelet-activating factor receptors located on surfaces of respiratory epithelial cells increases during viral infections. These receptors serve as attachment sites for pneumococci. Gram-negative organisms that are a part of gut flora also attach to specific receptors. Pili and adhesins on the microorganism surface play a pivotal role in this attachment. Pili were also shown to be important in the pathogenesis of sepsis caused by *Streptococcus pyogenes*, Group B streptococcus, and *S. pneumoniae* [9].

Bacteremia may ensue in patients whose defense mechanisms have become vulnerable due to many factors. The examples are as follows:

- With the intubation of an intensive care patient, protease activity increases whereas cell-bound fibronectin diminishes rendering cell surface receptors "sheathless," which make them ideal binding sites for predominantly Gram-negative bacteria of gut flora [9].

- Viridans streptococci, elements of oral flora, may cause bacteremia in neutropenic children who have severe oral mucositis and receiving antineoplastic chemotherapy.

- Gram-negative gut bacteria cause bacteremia by traversing the gut mucosa (translocation), whose integrity has been disrupted by antineoplastic drugs.

- Staphylococci, thanks to their ability to adhere to hard surfaces, cause catheter-related bacteremia by colonizing in catheter lumina.

4.2. The process of cytokine synthesis

The word "cytokine" is made up of two Greek words, "cyto-" (cell) and kinos (movement). The cytokine concept was introduced to scientific world by Barry Bloom and John David, who, being unaware of each other's similar research, discovered a cytokine, known as macrophage migration inhibitor factor today. Although cytokines were once classified as lymphokines, interleukins, and chemokines, according to their functions, and target and release sites, such a classification is avoided due to the abundance and substitution characteristics of cytokines [10].

Every cytokine has a corresponding cell surface receptor, with the stimulation of which begin signaling cascades, as a consequence of which some genes are upregulated or downregulated. In the end, either other cytokines or cell receptors for various molecules are synthesized, or the rate of synthesis of these substances decreases [10].

Sepsis and septic shock can be viewed as clinical pictures, which develop as consequences of pro-inflammatory processes/cytokines leading to a state that cannot be restrained by anti-inflammatory processes/cytokines (**Table 1**). The human body responds in a pathological manner to infection, which is a pathological situation itself. The occurrence of sepsis or immune compromise depends on whether systemic inflammatory response or its opposite end, compensatory anti-inflammatory response syndrome, predominates the inner environment as a response to infection. Compensatory anti-inflammatory response syndrome is a clinical entity, which progresses primarily with T-helper depression due to catecholamine discharge and apoptosis of splenic B-lymphocytes [11].

When the causative organism enters the body, nonspecific (innate) immune system is stimulated. Mammals perceive the pathogen by means of pattern-recognition receptors, the most important and evolutionally the oldest of which are Toll-like receptors (TLRs), found in insects, plants, and mammals. TLRs are transmembrane proteins, so-called because of their similarity to a product protein of the gene Toll, which is named after the remark ("Das ist ja toll!" ("That's really cool!")) by Nobel Prize in Physiology or Medicine winner (1995) Christina Nüsslein-Volhard, who has reportedly shouted out as so in surprise when she realized a *Drosophila melanogaster* (common fruit fly) had assumed an amazing appearance as a result of

Proinflammatory	Anti-inflammatory
TNF-α	IL-1Ra
IL1b, IL-2, IL-6, IL-8, IL-15	IL-4
Neutrophil elastase	IL-10
IFN-γ	IL-13
Thromboxane	Type II IL-1 receptor
Platelet-activating factor	Transforming growth factor-b
Vasoactive neuropeptides	Adrenaline
Phospholipase A$_2$	Soluble TNF-α receptors
Plasminogen activator inhibitor-1	Leukotriene B4-receptor antagonist
Prostaglandins	
Prostacyclin	
Free radicals	
Soluble adhesion molecules	
Tyrosine kinase	
Protein kinase	
H$_2$S	
NO	
High mobility group box 1 protein	

TNF: tumor necrosis factor, IL: interleukin, IFN: interferon.

Table 1. Major proinflammatory and anti-inflammatory mediators [12].

polymorphism of one of its proteins [13]. Transmembrane proteins have their extracellular, transmembrane, and intracellular parts. Humans have at least 10 different TLRs [14]. TLRs are found in abundance on leukocytes, macrophages, and some kinds of endothelial cells [11]. It is noteworthy that some TLRs are found on cytoplasmic membrane and some on the membrane of endocytic vesicles. These receptors recognize many organisms, from bacteria to fungi, and from protozoa to viruses. Although a part of nonspecific immune system, TLRs vary with respect to the patterns concerning the component of the organism they recognize. For instance, whereas TLR4 is unique in recognizing lipopolysaccharide of Gram-negative bacteria, mannan of *Candida albicans,* and glucuronoxylomannan of *Cryptococcus neoformans,* glycosylphosphatidylinositol moieties of *Plasmodium falciparum* are recognized by either TLR4 or TLR2. Hemozoin of *P. falciparum* is exclusively recognized by TLR9 [15].

Stimulated TLRs cause many protein kinases to be phosphorilized, in other words, become active. Reactions of these highly complex biochemical pathways take place in cytosol or endosome. Some of the biochemical pathways are dependent on a mediator molecule named MyD88, and some are not. For example, proinflammatory cytokines in sepsis and septic shock are released in a MyD88-dependent pathway. The end products of these pathways (nuclear factor kappa B ($NF_\kappa B$), interferon regulatory factor 3 (IRF3)) traverse the nuclear membrane and induce related genes by adhering to promotor regions of deoxyribonucleic acid (DNA). $Nf_\kappa B$ activity is inhibited by the most-studied heat-shock protein HSP70, which, thus, diminishes the inflammatory response. HSP70 reduces the damage caused by excessive inflammation by decreasing apoptosis and preserving cell proteins [16].

Significant information has been obtained with the study of inflammatory processes, especially those induced by Gram-negative bacteria. Septic shock occurs via similar mechanisms with Gram-positive organisms. Here, instead of lipopolysaccharide, which is found in abundance in Gram-negative organisms, less potent cell wall molecules, such as peptidoglycan and teicoic acid, cause similar inflammatory responses.

Gram-negative bacteria have a thin cell wall made up of a single layer of peptidoglycan, out of which there is a cell membrane consisting of lipopolysaccharide, which is a strong stimulator of immune response. The lipopolysaccharide molecule has three main components [17]:

1. **Lipid A** is responsible for the biological activity of endotoxin. Its structure is almost the same in different strains.

2. **Core polysaccharide** is made up of oligosaccharides, but its structure is highly diverse among species, even within strains.

3. **Oligosaccharide side chains** vary among strains. It consists of repeating units (e.g., 40 repetitions in O antigen) and is the moiety which provides the O antigen its antigenic specificity.

Lipopolysaccharide first binds to lipopolysaccharide-binding protein (LBP) in plasma. LBP-lipopolysaccharide complex binds to CD14 molecule on the plasma membrane. This new complex binds to TRL4/MD ("myeloid differentiating factor")-2, which is also on the plasma membrane [18]. This structure, activating various protein kinases, as outlined above, causes cytokine release when the end products bind to promotor regions on DNA [19].

There are countless cytokines playing roles in sepsis and septic shock. These mediators, causing release of each other, create an enormous mediator cascade. The mediator cascade is initiated by the stimulation of tumor necrosis factor (TNF) (cachectin) production by stimulators like lipopolysaccharide, C5a, viruses, and enterotoxins. TNF appears to be the main cytokine initiating and playing a pivotal role in the progression of the mediator cascade. TNF, released from many cells, such as monocytes, macrophages, natural killer cells, microglial cells, and hepatic Kupfer cells, causes countless mediators (e.g., interleukin(IL)-1β, IL-6, eicosanoids, platelet activation factor) to spill into blood in an uncontrolled manner resulting in a very severe inflammatory response and endothelial damage. However, there are many cytokines, the productions of which do not necessitate the presence of TNF [20]. As a consequence of this process, typical signs of endotoxic shock will show up. Some of the cytokines released (e.g., TNF-α, IL-1, and IL-6) cause free oxygen radical and protease release from other immune system cells, such as neutrophils, prostanoids leukotrienes, thromboxanes, nitric oxide, and endothelin from endothelial cells. Some of these substances are useful in killing bacteria but some (e.g., nitric oxide) are known to cause mitochondrial dysfunction by deactivating the catecholamines in the circulation. Mediators, whose release is induced by lipopolysaccharide, increase nitric oxide synthase II production and thus nitric oxide (endothelial-origin relaxation factor) production. Nitric oxide is a potent vasodilator and is the primary substance responsible for the hypotension in septic shock. Besides, nitric oxide causes vasodilation, which in turn causes diminished perfusion pressure in capillary network and blood flow by opening collateral channels. Decreased capillary flow results in organ hypoxia despite high blood flow because of vasodilation.

We have enough knowledge on how sepsis and septic shock develop, but it is surprising that only a few histopathologic changes concerning cell death are present in patients who have died of severe sepsis. Apart from cellular apoptosis in spleen and intestines, myopathic changes in skeletal muscle, and changes in vascular morphology in meningococcal sepsis, there is no serious sign of necrosis in main organs.

Then, studies have concentrated on microcirculation and mitochondrial dysfunction, and theories on how adenosine triphosphate (ATP) production can decrease under normal, even supranormal oxygen partial pressures, have been put forward. These theories include diminished pyruvate entry into tricarboxylic acid cycle, activation of poly-(ADP-ribose) polymerase, and uncoupling of oxidation from phosphorylation. Another cause of tissue hypoxia is nitric oxide's combining with free oxygen radicals (O_2^-) to form peroxynitrite ($ONOO^-$) resulting in reversible or irreversible binding of these three substances to proteins in the electron transport chain, such as succinate dehydrogenase and cytochrome c oxidase. As a result, ATP production decreases, being unable to meet the needs of the energy-consuming cell, and cell death takes place. This process accounts for the unexpectedly few histopathologic changes in autopsies. Complement system is activated through contact with bacterial molecules or binding of proteins, such as antibody or mannose-binding lectin, to these molecules. Complements like C3b and C5a cause migration of leukocytes and increase inflammation [11].

The balance between thrombogenesis and thrombolysis has been disrupted in sepsis. There is endothelial damage due to direct effect of microorganisms, cytokines, and fibrin deposition triggered by endothelial dysfunction. As a result of this, a process of simultaneous thromboses and bleedings, which is known as consumption coagulopathy or disseminated intravascular coagulation (DIC), develops. DIC is more frequently encountered in Gram-negative sepsis (e.g., meningococcal sepsis) than in Gram-positive sepsis. The most common complications of DIC are thromboses of great vessels, liver infarction, acute renal failure, cerebral hemorrhage, and cerebral infarction [21].

4.3. Cytokines as sepsis biomarkers

TNF, IL-1b, and IL-6 are the first cytokines to regulate the initial response of the innate immune system. TNF and IL-1b activate endothelial cells and attract the granulocytes in circulation to inflammation site. TNF and IL-1b cause fever and other systemic signs by entering the circulation. IL-6 increases the production of what is known as acute phase proteins (e.g., C-reactive protein) in liver and more granulocytes in bone marrow. As can easily be seen, TNF, IL-1b, and IL-6 are responsible for the formation of SIRS and could be thought of being used as sepsis biomarkers [22].

TNF and IL-1b concentrations increase in endotoxin-associated Gram-negative sepsis. TNF or IL-1b administration to laboratory animals is as effective in the formation of septic shock as the endotoxin itself, but in clinical studies, TNF and IL-1b could not be used as sepsis biomarkers because

- TNF concentrations before anti-TNF antibody treatment do not affect the outcome.
- IL-1b does not rise as TNF does.

Of the three cytokines mentioned above, IL-6 has attracted the most attention. The causes of this include

- The role of IL-1b, IL-1a, and the receptor antagonist of IL-1 in the development of sepsis is debated [22].
- The relatively higher reliability of measurement of the plasma concentration of IL-6.
- The usability of IL-6 in the diagnosis and treatment of autoimmune rheumatologic diseases.
- The availability of commercial immunoassay kits, contrary to TNF and IL-1b.

Nevertheless exactly as in TNF and IL-1b, IL-6 is not specific to sepsis and its role as sepsis biomarker is prognostic, rather than diagnostic. In many studies, rise in IL-6 concentration is associated with higher mortality. This characteristic can be used to detect patients who may benefit from therapy [22].

Since the clinical signs of sepsis in neonates are very subtle and nonspecific, predictive biomarkers are needed, particularly in economically developing countries, where the incidence, morbidity, and mortality of early neonatal sepsis (ENS) (sepsis diagnosed less than 72 h after birth) are particularly high. Evidence published to date is still far from convincing the physician to use procalcitonin as a biomarker for routine use in clinical practice as a risk stratifier and a prognostic predictor or even to guide the duration of antibiotic treatment and bedside decision making [23]. The results of a new study by He et al. indicate that elevated IL-27 strongly correlates with ENS and may provide additional diagnostic value along with procalcitonin [24].

The usage of IL-6 and LBP in pediatrics is also promising. In newborns with late sepsis risk, IL-6 rises 48 h before bacterial sepsis becomes clinically manifest [25]. Initial high IL-6 concentrations predict future septic shock in hospitalized children [26]. Initial high IL-6 concentrations foretell high risk of septic shock and mortality in pediatric burn patients [27]. LBP points to invasive bacterial infections and bacterial infections in children and newborns over 28 weeks of gestational age, respectively [28–30]. LBP can differentiate between SIRS and ENS in newborns within the first 48 h of their lives [30].

While homing chemokines serve to regulate adaptive immune system, especially in secondary lymphoid tissue, proinflammatory chemokines attract granulocytes and monocytes to the site of inflammation and promote their extravasation. Chemokines, thanks to these properties, can be used as biomarkers in sepsis, and some of them have been shown to be superior to IL-6 in that aspect. Examples are IL-8 (in the diagnosis of sepsis) and monocyte chemoattractant protein (MCP)-1 (in the determination of sepsis mortality) [31]. According to the results of a study, among 17 cytokines (IL-1β, IL-2, IL-4, IL-5, IL-6, IL-7, IL-8, IL-10, IL-12, IL-13, IL-17, interferon-γ, granulocyte colony-stimulating factor, granulocyte-macrophage colony-stimulating factor, MCP-1, macrophage inflammatory protein-1, and TNF-α), the cytokines most closely associated with organ dysfunction within 24 h are IL-8 and MCP-1 [31]. As yet, a cytokine which is uniquely associated with severe sepsis and septic shock and can be used as a biomarker has not been discovered [32].

4.4. Effect of cytokine storm on tissues and organs

- Cardiovascular system

    Myocardium is depressed in septic shock. The reason for this depression is not hypoperfusion, but depressing cytokines like TNF and IL-1β in the circulation. Ventricules dilate and ejection fraction drops. As a result, hypoperfusion ensues in peripheral tissues. Peripheral hypoperfusion and hypoxia lead to overproduction of lactic acid, which is another myocardial depressor. This chain of events persists as a vicious cycle [21].

- Respiratory system

    Alveoli are diffusely damaged because of circulating endotoxins. In the exudative phase of this damage, proteinaceous edema fluid accumulates in alveoli, and type I epithelial cells are injured. In this clinical picture, which is also known as shock lung, alveolar collapse, hemorrhage, edema, hyaline membrane formation, which is made up of fibrin and necrotic epithelial cells on epithelial surfaces of respiratory bronchioles and alveolar ducti, and neutrophil accumulation in alveolar capillaries occur. Unless treated, severe pulmonary edema develops despite low central venous pressure, and as a result, ventilation-perfusion mismatch ensues. This clinical picture is called ARDS. In the regeneration phase, healing occurs via return to normal structure or pulmonary fibrosis. Lost type 1 cells are replaced by proliferating type 2 cells. Superimposing infections and barotrauma due to mechanical ventilation worsen respiratory system functions [21].

- Kidneys

    Nitric oxide disrupts blood distribution in renal medulla and cortex. With the effect of nitric oxide and cytokines, renal tubule function, which requires high energy input, deteriorates due to decreasing ATP production. As a consequence of hypotension, increase in the release of endothelin, which is a vasopressor hormone, and activation of renin-angiotensin-aldosterone system pave the way to sodium and water retention, which makes a ground for renal failure. Neutrophil adhesion and microthrombi further diminish the glomerular filtration rate. The question of why renal failure in sepsis, despite anuria and despite its presence even in patients who die of sepsis, can develop without acute tubular necrosis and why it takes renal function so long (months) to return to normal while systemic inflammation has already disappeared and circulatory function has returned to normal still stands as an enigma and awaits to be elucidated [11, 21].

- Central and peripheral nervous system

    The most important one among the effects of sepsis on central nervous system is sepsis-related encephalopathy and critical illness polyneuropathy. The causes of encephalopathy include disruption of blood-brain barrier, coagulopathy-related cerebral hemorrhage, microinfarctions, hypoxic-ischemic encephalopathy, metastatic brain abscesses, meningitis, and cytokine storm. While this clinical entity, which manifest itself with delirium and confusion, is often reversible, it may lead to self-mutilism of the patient in intensive care and development of cognitive and behavioral dysfunction in the long term.

    The diagnosis of this clinical picture, which manifests itself also with flaccid paralysis and loss of deep tendon reflexes, is usually made only during or after separation of the patient from ventilator due to encephalopathy, administration of neuromuscular drugs, and the unfavorable general situation of the patient. Prognosis varies according to the severity of illness and patient's age. Muscle weakness may last for months [21].

- Gastrointestinal system

    Gastrointestinal system is negatively affected by sepsis due to hypoperfusion. Gastrointestinal bleeding may ensue as a consequence of splanchnic hypoperfusion, increase in intestinal permeability, bacterial translocation, stress ulcers, and coagulopathy.

    Although liver is relatively resistant to sepsis, transaminase elevation, peribiliary infarctions, and cholestatic jaundice may ensue as a result of hypotension [21].

- Immune system

    Although an immunologic hyperreaction itself, sepsis further disrupts the integrity of the immune system. In survivors of sepsis, mortality rate is higher in the following several years than that in normal population, which can be attributed to a vague immune disorder with cytokines and chemokines [21, 33]. Overproduction of anti-inflammatory cytokines may be a cause of immune deficiency in sepsis, but there is no evidence that the abundance of anti-inflammatory cytokines (such as IL-1 receptor antagonist and soluble TNF receptors) in the environment is sufficient for putting away the effects of proinflammatory cytokines [20].

- Extremities

    A clinical picture of skin bleeding and necrosis due to microvascular thrombi and subsequent perivascular hemorrhage may develop, especially in the presence of disseminated intravascular coagulation. This is called purpura fulminans (PF). Although most frequently encountered in N. meningitidis bacteremia, PF may ensue in bloodstream infections due to S. pneumoniae and capsulated microorganisms of any kind. In addition to necroses in PF, vasoconstriction in sepsis may be severe enough to cause infarctions of fingers and autoamputation. Vasopressor drugs, if administered without fluid resuscitation, increase the risk for this complication [21, 33].

- Mental status

    Psychological disorders, such as posttraumatic stress disorder (in 20% of ARDS patients), depression, panic attack, public isolation, inability to stay alone or in crowded areas, and decrease in sexual activity, are seen frequently in survivors of sepsis [21].

4.5. The role of gene polymorphisms in predisposition to sepsis

Whether there is an association between the severity of sepsis and septic shock and cytokine gene polymorphisms is an important field of study. Such a connection could not be shown with IL-1, IL-1 receptor antagonist, and IL-10 genes. It has been postulated that TNF2, being a rare TNF gene (adenine at −308 position), may be associated with high promoter activity, but no elevation in the prevalence of TNF2 allele in patients having frequent attacks of severe sepsis and infections due to Gram-negative organisms has been noted. There is a publication stating that rare Arg753Gln mutation of TLR2 renders individuals prone to staphylococcal sepsis [33]. Single-nucleotide polymorphism in IL-1β gene was found associated with higher mortality [34].

5. Medical history

In sepsis, complaints leading to the child being brought to the physician vary according to the source of infection or SIRS. Fever, hypothermia tachypnea, stomach ache, vomiting, diarrhea, clouding of consciousness, or several of these may be present in the child. Features in the history such as the child's immunization status, past infections, and attending daycare should be taken into notice [35].

6. Physical examination

Fever or hypothermia (core body temperature <36°C) may be observed [5]. Abnormalities in other vital signs may also be detected. Normal limits of vital signs according to age are depicted in **Table 2** [36].

Shock may not be present in sepsis. Hypotension is not a prerequisite for shock. Mottled skin and prolongation of capillary refill time may help the physician recognize septic shock before hypotension emerges [2, 5].

Age group	Bradycardia (pulse/min)	Tachycardia (pulse/min)	Respiratory rate (respirations/min)	Systolic blood pressure (mmHg)
0 day to 1 week	<100	<180	>50	<65
1 week to 1 month	<100	<180	>40	<75
1 month to 1 year	<90	<180	>34	<100
2–5 years	<80	<140	>22	<94
6–12 years	<70	<130	>18	<105
13–18 years	<60	<110	>14	<117

Table 2. Normal of vital signs according to age [36].

7. Laboratory tests

In a child suspected of having sepsis, the following tests may be ordered: complete blood count (always with differentials), a reasonable metabolic panel (electrolytes, glucose, liver function tests, and albumin), serum lactate, arterial blood gases, coagulation studies, amylase, lipase, urinalysis, sputum culture, and Gram stain [35]. Leukocytosis or leukopenia may be present in children with sepsis (**Table 3**) [2].

Antibiotics should be started after blood and other cultures being drawn unless a delay of longer than 45 min is expected because of this process. According to the results of a recent study, the diagnosis of pediatric septicemia through BACTEC 9240 is quicker with high yield and great sensitivity compared to the conventional technique [37]. Blood cultures are recommended to be taken from a peripheral vein and a catheter, which has been in place for more than 48 h into a set of aerobic and anaerobic bottles and as at least two sets. In case the volume of the blood is insufficient, the sensitivity of the blood culture will decrease, and vice versa [38, 39]. The author suggests that anaerobic blood cultures not be taken from children routinely, since

- The volume of blood that can be taken from children is limited.
- True anaerobic blood stream infections are rare (<5%) in children.
- Instead of sets consisting of one aerobic and one anaerobic bottle, selective culture for anaerobic organisms with two aerobic bottles yields better results (6% more positives).

- Since sensitivity patterns of anaerobes are well known, they can be covered effectively with empirical therapy.

Age group	Leukocyte count ($\times 10^3/\mu L$)
0–7 days	>34
1 week to 1 month	>19.5 or <5
1 month to 1 year	>17.5 or <5
2–5 years	>15.5 or <6
6–12 years	>13.5 or <4.5
12–18 years	>11 or <4.5

Table 3. Leukocyte counts according to age [2].

Even if anaerobic blood cultures are to be drawn, the indications should be limited to risky situations as below [40–42]:

- Children displaying abnormal abdominal symptoms and signs.
- Children with sacral decubitus ulcers or cellulitis.
- Patients with poor oral hygiene, severe oral mucositis, or chronic sinusitis.
- Neutropenic children receiving high-dose corticosteroid therapy, which may mask abdominal symptoms.
- Children with sickle cell disease.
- Infants of mothers with prolonged rupture of membranes or chorioamnionitis.
- Children thought to have bacteremia due to a human bite or crushing trauma.

When clinically indicated, cultures may be taken from urine, cerebrospinal fluid, wounds, respiratory secretions, and other body fluids. Most accurate results will probably be obtained with double quantitative blood cultures in case of an intravascular device-related bloodstream infection. Mannan, antimannan, and 1,3 beta-D-glucan tests may be used if invasive candidiasis is suspected. Imaging techniques are very useful to delineate the foci of infection and to decide whether the patient's condition is suitable for transport [5].

8. Diagnosis and differential diagnosis

Risk-scoring systems may guide the physician in deciding the presence of a serious bacterial infection [43]. As mentioned above, if a probable or proven infection is present with SIRS, the child is in sepsis. Sepsis should be differentiated from other causes of SIRS (e.g., trauma, burn, acute pancreatitis, drug reaction (acetaminophen, cytarabine, IL-2)) and hypotension (e.g., hypovolemic shock, cardiogenic shock, neurogenic shock, and adrenocortical insufficiency) [4, 44–46]. The value of procalcitonin and other biomarkers in the differential diagnosis of sepsis is under investigation [5].

9. Management

The management of severe sepsis and septic shock involves the following phases:

9.1. Hemodynamic support

Hemodynamic support should be started promptly without waiting for the intensive care admission. A protocol on recognizing septic shock in emergency ward may shorten the time that is passed for the initiation of appropriate therapy [47]. Although central venous line is preferred, fluids may be given through peripheral veins or via intraosseous route if a central venous catheter is not present or cannot be placed [5, 48]. Initial recommended fluid is crystalloid (e.g., normal saline) in boli of 20 mL/kg, each administered in 5–10 min. It should be kept in mind that mortality in children may be reduced if albumin is used in the initial fluid [49]. These crystalloids or colloid boli are continued until the perfusion returns to normal and the total given fluid volume reaches 60 mL/kg or more unless hepatomegaly or rales develop [48]. It is imperative that fluid resuscitation be given as rapidly as possible and not sparingly. The mortality in children who were given a total of more than 40 mL/kg is about 40% lower than those given a total of less than 20 mL/kg. The duration of intensive care and hospital stay become shorter (2–3 days) in patients given 60 mL/kg of fluid in the first 60 min than those who are not [50–52]. Inotropic support is recommended instead of fluid replacement if hepatomegaly or crackles are present. If the child has severe hemolytic anemia and blood pressure is normal, blood transfusion should be preferred to crystalloid or albumin boli [5].

For children in respiratory distress or hypoxia, oxygen should be administered with a mask; thereafter, if needed and if possible, high-flow oxygen through nasal cannula or nasopharyngeal continuous positive air pressure (CPAP) may be carried out [5, 48]. An adequate cardiovascular resuscitation reduces the likelihood of cardiovascular instability if mechanical ventilation is needed [5].

In the early management (in the first hour and in emergency ward), clinical goals for the septic shock patient are the following:

- Bring the capillary refill time back to 2 s or less.
- Provide blood pressure normal for age.
- Obtain a normal pulse and heart rate by removing the difference between central and peripheral pulses.
- Warm the extremities.
- Raise the urine output above 1 mL/kg/h.

- Restore hypoglycemia and hypocalcemia back to normal.
- Restore mental status.

Antibiotics should have been started meanwhile [5, 48, 53].

Goals to be realized by invasive monitorization of the patient are as follows:

- Central venous oxygen saturation of 70% or above and
- Cardiac index of 3.3–6 L/min/m² [5, 54]

9.2. Inotropes, vasopressors, and vasodilators

The patients whose initial fluid therapy has been completed in 10–15 min and who are unresponsive to this therapy (twice crystalloid or colloid boli) should have been started inotrope support at about 15th min of management through a peripheral vein if necessary until central venous route is assured [5, 55]. The goals at this stage of the management are as follows [5]:

- Normal perfusion pressure (mean arterial pressure, central venous pressure): 55 mmHg for term newborns, 60 mmHg for children 1 month to 1 year of age, 65 mmHg for children aged 1–15 years.
- Central venous oxygen saturation ($ScvO_2$) = 70%.
- Cardiac index = 3.3–6 L/min/m².

In cold shock with normal blood pressure but abnormal capillary refill time (>2 s), the dosage of dopamine given through central vein can be increased to 10 µg/kg/min. If shock is refractory to dopamine, epinephrine (0.05–3 µg/kg/min) should be given; $ScvO_2$ and hemoglobin (Hb) should be kept above 70% and 10 g/dL, respectively. If $ScvO_2$ persists below 70%, a vasodilator, such as milrinone and imrinone, should be added to therapy; levosimendan should be considered to be started [5, 48].

In cold shock with low blood pressure, $ScvO_2$ and Hb should be kept above 70% and 10 g/dL, respectively. If shock is refractory to dopamine, epinephrine (0.05–3 µg/kg/min) should be given; if hypotension persists, norepinephrine should be started. If $ScvO_2$ is still below 70%, dobutamine, milrinone, enoksimone, or levosimendan should be considered [5, 48].

In warm shock with low blood pressure, the rate of norepinephrine should be adjusted such that $ScvO_2$ stays above 70%. If hypotension persists, vasopressin, terlipressin, or angiotensin should be considered. If $ScvO_2$ is still below 70%, low-dose epinephrine should be considered [5, 48].

In some patients, in whom systemic vascular resistance is very low despite norepinephrine administration, vasopressin, and terlipressin were used, but no benefit from these drugs has been shown in randomized studies [56–60]. In patients with low cardiac output, but high systemic vascular resistance, vasodilators such as

- Calcium sensitizer (levosimendan).
- Type III phosphodiesterase inhibitors (amrinone, enoximone, or milrinone).

- Nitrovasodilators.
- Prostacyclin.
- Fenoldopam.
- Pentoxifylline.

have been proposed in addition to inotropes [5].

If no response is taken with this therapy, the case is accepted as catecholamine-resistant shock, and the patient should be started hydrocortisone if at risk for absolute adrenal insufficiency [5, 48].

If catecholamine-resistant shock persists, pneumothorax, pericardial effusion, and high intraabdominal pressure should be excluded or corrected if present; pulmonary artery catheter, pulse contour cardiac output catheter, and femoral artery thermodilution catheter should be used or Doppler ultrasonography should be considered to receive some guidance on therapy [48].

If, despite all these measures, shock cannot be taken under control, extracorporeal membrane oxygenation (ECMO) should be considered [5, 61, 62].

9.3. Antimicrobial therapy

After severe sepsis is recognized, antibiotics should be started in the first hour, even in the first 15 min if possible. Cultures should be taken before initializing therapy if feasible, but therapy should not be delayed for this reason. The choice of antibiotic should be in accordance with endemic or epidemic data. Intramuscular or oral route may be used until intravenous access is made. In toxic shock syndromes with refractory hypotension, clindamycin and antitoxin are recommended. The management of *Clostridium difficile* colitis is preferentially carried out with enteral antibiotics; vancomycin should be used for severe colitis. Antimicrobial therapy should continually be reevaluated with regard to deescalation [5].

Combination empirical therapy is recommended for neutropenic patients with severe sepsis and in places where difficult-to-treat organisms, such as Acinetobacter and Pseudomonas, are prevalent. This therapy should be in the form of a wide-spectrum beta-lactam antibiotic + an aminoglycoside/quinolone in places where the risk of infection due to Pseudomonas is high. If the prevalence of *S. pneumoniae* is high, a beta-lactam + macrolide combination is recommended. Combination therapy should be of short duration (3–5 days or less) according to antibiotic-sensitivity results [5].

The duration of antimicrobial therapy should be limited to 7–10 days unless

- The response is slow,
- The infection focus is undrainable,
- *S. aureus* bacteremia is present,
- Some fungus or virus infections are present,

- An immunologic disorder with neutropenia is present, or

- Pneumonia due to *Pseudomonas spp.* or other Gram-negative rods is present [5, 63].

Narrowing the antimicrobial spectrum and shortening the duration of antimicrobial therapy would prevent superinfections due to other agents, such as *Candida* spp., *C. difficile*, and vancomycin-resistant *Enterococcus faecium* [5].

Antiviral therapy should be started in sepsis or septic shock due to viruses. Antimicrobial therapy should be stopped in case that the cause of sepsis was detected as something other than infection. The removal of infected intravascular devices, especially central venous catheters, if possible and if preferred to antibiotic lock methods, will reduce mortality and increase the chances that the infection will be cured [5, 64].

9.4. Transfusions

If superior vena cava oxygen saturation is low (<70%), Hb concentration should be maintained at 10 g/dL. After hypoxemia and shock subside, the goal for Hb should be over 7 g/dL. Higher concentrations may be needed if acute bleeding, severe hypoxemia, or ischemic heart disease is present [5, 65, 66].

Platelet transfusion is indicated if the platelet count is

- Below 10,000/μL without a detectable bleeding.

- Below 20,000/μL if the patient has significant bleeding risk.

- Below 50,000/μL in the presence of active bleeding or in situations requiring either surgical or invasive procedures.

Plasma therapy should be brought to the agenda in case of thrombotic purpura situations, such as progressive disseminated intravascular coagulation due to sepsis, secondary thrombotic microangiopathy, and thrombotic thrombocytopenic purpura. In the absence of planned invasive intervention or bleeding, antithrombin therapy, erythropoietin administration for sepsis-associated anemia, and fresh-frozen plasma therapy should be avoided.

9.5. Corticosteroids

Hydrocortisone should be given to children with severe sepsis only in the presence of suspected or proven adrenal insufficiency, because there are publications both favoring (for reduction in mortality) and discouraging (for increasing mortality) its use [5, 67, 68]. Risk factors for adrenal insufficiency include severe septic shock with purpura, steroid use for chronic illness, and hypophysis or adrenal gland abnormalities. Hydrocortisone infusion is started with the dosage of 50 mg/m^2/24, which may be needed to be increased up to 50 mg/kg/day in a short time. The measurement of baseline serum cortisol concentration may be useful at the onset of therapy [5].

9.6. Miscellaneous recommendations

In ARDS, tidal volumes exceeding 10 mL/kg should be avoided. Plateau pressure, arterial pH, and arterial partial oxygen pressure should be maintained at 30 cmH$_2$O or below, between 7.3–7.45 and 60–80 Torr (8–10.7 kPa), respectively. The Hb goal of 10 g/dL in unstable patients should be taken as 7 g/dL after recovery from shock and deep hypoxia [69].

Water retention in patients recovering from shock should be treated with diuretics. If this fails, continuous venovenous hemofiltration or intermittent dialysis should be carried out in order to prevent water retention of more than 10% of the body weight [5].

In children with septic shock, glucose concentration should be maintained below 180 mg/dL since concentrations of 178 mg/dL and over are associated with higher mortality. In newborns and children, insulin therapy should be given along with glucose infusion, the rate of which should be 4–6 mg/kg/min (6–8 mg/kg/min in newborns). The alternative is giving maintenance fluids prepared with 10% dextrose in water [5, 70].

Although no sedative or sedation protocol is recommended for patients with sepsis and mechanical ventilation support, long-term propofol should be avoided in children below 3 years for its association with fatal metabolic acidosis. Etodomidate and dexmedetomidine should also be avoided due to its inhibitory effect on adrenal axis and sympathetic nervous system, the integrity of which is essential for hemodynamic stability in septic shock [5].

Enteral route should be preferred to parenteral route in nutrition. Glucose requirements of newborns and children can be met with sodium-containing fluids prepared with 10% dextrose in water and administered at maintenance rate.

10. Prognosis

Hospital mortality of pediatric sepsis is 2–10% [5]. In United States, hospital mortality in severe sepsis has declined from 10% in 1995 to 4% in 2003 [71, 72]; this is probably because septic shock is increasingly recognized more readily and earlier in the course and treated more aggressively [73].

Seven and six percent of children who are discharged from hospital after surviving postneonatal sepsis die within 28 days and afterward, respectively (early and late mortality). About half of those who survive these 28 days are rehospitalized at least once. Comorbidity is important in the development and late mortality of and rehospitalization in pediatric sepsis [74, 75].

11. Conclusion

As sepsis in children continues to take lives of children, especially in economically developing countries, it will continue to be the focus of attention for physicians, scientists, and the public. Although there are a few newer antibiotics in the pipeline, other novel therapies hold promise for overcoming this "cytokine storm disease" in near future.

Author details

Selim Öncel

Address all correspondence to: selimOncel@doctor.com

Division of Pediatric Infectious Diseases, Department of Pediatrics and Child Health, Section of Internal Medical Sciences, Kocaeli University Faculty of Medicine, Kocaeli, Turkey

References

[1] Sepsis Alliance. Sepsis and Children [Internet]. 2017. Available from: http://www.sepsis.org/sepsis-and/children/[Accessed: 2017-02-05].

[2] Goldstein B, Giroir B, Randolph A, International Consensus Conference on Pediatric Sepsis. International pediatric sepsis consensus conference: definitions for sepsis and organ dysfunction in pediatrics. Pediatr Crit Care Med. 2005;6:2-8. DOI: 10.1097/01.PCC.0000149131.72248.E6

[3] Lever A, Mackenzie I. Sepsis: definition, epidemiology, and diagnosis. BMJ. 2007;335:879-883. DOI: 10.1136/bmj.39346.495880.AE

[4] Martin GS. Sepsis, severe sepsis and septic shock: changes in incidence, pathogens and outcomes. Expert Rev Anti Infect Ther. 2012;10:701-6. DOI: 10.1586/eri.12.50

[5] Dellinger RP, Levy MM, Rhodes A, Annane D, Gerlach H, Opal SM, et al. Surviving Sepsis Campaign: international guidelines for management of severe sepsis and septic shock, 2012. Intensive Care Med. 2013;39:165-228. DOI: 10.1007/s00134-012-2769-8

[6] Laupland KB, Gregson DB, Vanderkooi OG, Ross T, Kellner JD. The changing burden of pediatric bloodstream infections in Calgary, Canada, 2000-2006. Pediatr Infect Dis J. 2009;28:114-117. DOI: 10.1097/INF.0b013e318187ad5a

[7] Watson RS, Carcillo J. Scope and epidemiology of pediatric sepsis. Pediatr Crit Care Med. 2005;6(3 Suppl):S3-5. DOI: 0.1097/01.PCC.0000161289.22464.C3

[8] Tibby S, Nadel S, Paolo, Arenas-Lopez S, Ewald U, Härtel C, et al. Report on the expert meeting on neonatal and paediatric sepsis. European Medicines Agency [Internet]. 2010.

Available from: http://www.ema.europa.eu/docs/en_GB/document_library/Report/2010/12/WC500100199.pdf [Accessed: 2017-02-05]

[9] Kaplan SL, Vallejo JG. Bacteremia and septic shock. In: Feigin RD, Cherry JD, Demmler-Harrison GJ, Kaplan SL, editors. Feigin & Cherry's Textbook of Pediatric Infectious Diseases. 6th ed. Philadelphia: Saunders Elsevier; 2009. p. 837-851.

[10] Wikipedia contributors. Cytokine. Wikipedia, The Free Encyclopedia [Internet]. 2013. Available from: http://en.wikipedia.org/wiki/Cytokine [Accessed: 2017-02-05]

[11] Mitchell E, Whitehouse T. The pathophysiology of sepsis. In: Daniels R, Nutbeam T, editors. ABC of Sepsis. 1st ed. West Sussex: Blackwell Publishing Ltd; 2010. p. 20-24.

[12] Ramnath RD, Weing S, He M, Sun J, Zhang H, Manmish Singh B, et al. Inflammatory mediators in sepsis: Cytokines, chemokines, adhesion molecules and gases. J Org Dysfunct. 2006;2:80-92. DOI: 10.1080/17471060500435662

[13] O'Neill LAJ, Brint E, editors. Toll-like Receptors in Inflammation. 1st ed. Basel: Birkhäuser Verlag; 2005.

[14] Takeda K, Yamamoto M, Honda K. Assessing the response of cells to TLR stimulation. In: Konat GW, editor. Signaling by Toll-like Receptors. 1st ed. Boca Raton: CRC Press; 2008. p. 1-22.

[15] Uematsu S, Akira S. Toll-like receptors (TLRs) and their ligands. In: Bauer S, Hartmann G, editörler. Toll-Like Receptors (TLRs) and Innate Immunity. 1st ed. Heidelberg: Springer-Verlag; 2008. p. 1-20.

[16] Bromberg Z, Weiss YG, Deutschman CS. Heat shock proteins in inflammation. In: Abraham E, Singer M, editors. Mechanisms of Sepsis-Induced Organ Dysfunction and Recovery. 1st ed. Heidelberg: Springer-Verlag Berlin Heidelberg; 2007. p. 113-121.

[17] Silipo A, Molinaro A. The diversity of the core oligosaccharide in lipopolysaccharides. In: Wang X, Quinn PJ, editörler. Endotoxins: Structure, Function and Recognition. 1st ed. Dordrecht: Springer; 2010. p. 69-99.

[18] Gangloff M, Gay NJ. MD-2: the Toll "gatekeeper" in endotoxin signalling. Trends Biochem. Sci. 2004;29:294-300. DOI: 10.1016/j.tibs.2004.04.008

[19] Hoebe K, Beutler B. TLRs as bacterial sensors. In: O'Neill LAJ, Brint E, editors. Toll-like Receptors in Inflammation. 1st ed. Basel: Birkhäuser Verlag; 2005. p. 1-17.

[20] Cavaillon J-M, Adib-Conquy M, Fitting C, Adrie C, Payen D. Cytokine cascade in sepsis. Scand J Infect Dis. 2003;35:535-544. DOI: 10.1080/00365540310015935

[21] Cilliers H, Whitehouse T, Tunnicliffe B. Serious complications of sepsis. In: Daniels R, Nutbeam T, editors. ABC of Sepsis. 1st ed. West Sussex: Blackwell Publishing Ltd; 2010. p. 15-19.

[22] Faix JD. Biomarkers of sepsis. Crit Rev Clin Lab Sci. 2013;50:23-36. DOI: 10.3109/10408363.2013.764490

[23] Lanziotti VS, Póvoa P, Soares M, Silva JR, Barbosa AP, Salluh JI. Use of biomarkers in pediatric sepsis: literature review. Rev Bras Ter Intensiva. 2016;28:472-482. DOI: 10.5935/0103-507X.20160080

[24] He Y, Du WX, Jiang HY, Ai Q, Feng J, Liu Z, Yu JL. Multiplex cytokine profiling identifies interleukin-27 as a novel biomarker for neonatal early onset sepsis. Shock. 2017;47:140-147. DOI: 10.1097/SHK.0000000000000753

[25] Küster H, Weiss M, Willeitner AE, Detlefsen S, Jeremias I, Zbojan J, et al. Interleukin-1 receptor antagonist and interleukin-6 for early diagnosis of neonatal sepsis 2 days before clinical manifestation. Lancet. 1998;352:1271-1277. DOI: 10.1016/S0140-6736(98)08148-3

[26] Fioretto JR, Martin JG, Kurokawa CS, Carpi MF, Bonatto RC, Ricchetti SMQ, et al. Interleukin-6 and procalcitonin in children with sepsis and septic shock. Cytokine. 2008;43:160-164. DOI: 10.1016/j.cyto.2008.05.005

[27] Finnerty CC, Herndon DN, Chinkes DL, Jeschke MG. Serum cytokine differences in severely burned children with and without sepsis. Shock. 2007;27:4-9. DOI: 10.1097/01.shk.0000235138.20775.36

[28] Behrendt D, Dembinski J, Heep A, Bartmann P. Lipopolysaccharide binding protein in preterm infants. Arch Dis Child Fetal Neonatal Ed. 2004;89:F551-554. DOI: 10.1136/adc.2003.030049

[29] Ubenauf KM, Krueger M, Henneke P, Berner R. Lipopolysaccharide binding protein is a potential marker for invasive bacterial infections in children. Pediatr Infect Dis J. 2007;26:159-162. DOI: 10.1097/01.inf.0000253064.88722.6d

[30] Pavcnik-Arnol M, Hojker S, Derganc M. Lipopolysaccharide-binding protein in critically ill neonates and children with suspected infection: comparison with procalcitonin, interleukin-6, and C-reactive protein. Intensive Care Med. 2004;30:1454-1460. DOI: 10.1007/s00134-004-2307-4

[31] Bozza FA, Salluh JI, Japiassu AM, Soares M, Assis EF, Gomes RN, et al. Cytokine profiles as markers of disease severity in sepsis: a multiplex analysis. Crit Care. 2007;11:R49. DOI: 10.1186/cc5783

[32] Lvovschi V, Arnaud L, Parizot C, Freund Y, Juillien G, Ghillani-Dalbin P, et al. Cytokine profiles in sepsis have limited relevance for stratifying patients in the emergency department: a prospective observational study. PLoS One. 2011;6:e28870. DOI: 10.1371/journal.pone.0028870

[33] Munford RS, Suffredini AF. Sepsis, severe sepsis, and septic shock. In: Mandell GL, Bennett JE, Dolin R, editors. Mandell, Douglas, and Bennett's Principles and Practice of Infectious Diseases. Philadelphia: Churchill Livingstone Elsevier; 2010. p. 987-1010.

[34] Stüber F. Cytokine gene polymorphism and host susceptibility to infection. In: Kotb M, Calandra T, editors. Cytokines and Chemokines in Infectious Diseases Handbook. 1st ed. Totowa: Humana Press Inc.; 2003. p. 23-30.

[35] DynaMed Editorial Team. Sepsis in children [Internet]. DynaMed [database online]. 2017 [updated: 2013 Jan 26; cited: 2017 Feb 05]. Available from: http://www.ebscohost.com/dynamed

[36] Fleming S, Thompson M, Stevens R, Heneghan C, Plüddemann A, Maconochie I, et al. Normal ranges of heart rate and respiratory rate in children from birth to 18 years of age: a systematic review of observational studies. Lancet. 2011;**377**:1011-1018. DOI: 10.1016/S0140-6736(10)62226-X

[37] Ahmad A, Iram S, Hussain S, Yusuf NW. Diagnosis of paediatric sepsis by automated blood culture system and conventional blood culture. J Pak Med Assoc. 2017;**67**:192-195. PMID: 28138169

[38] Connell TG, Rele M, Cowley D, Buttery JP, Curtis N. How reliable is a negative blood culture result? Volume of blood submitted for culture in routine practice in a children's hospital. Pediatrics. 2007;**119**:891-896. DOI: 10.1542/peds.2006-0440

[39] Isaacman DJ, Karasic RB, Reynolds EA, Kost SI. Effect of number of blood cultures and volume of blood on detection of bacteremia in children. J Pediatr. 1996;**128**:190-195. PMID: 8636810

[40] Morris AJ, ilson ML, Mirrett S, Reller LB. Rationale for selective use of anaerobic blood cultures. J Clin Microbiol. 1993;**31**:2110-2113. PMCID: PMC265706

[41] Zaidi AK, Knaut AL, Mirrett S, Reller LB. Value of routine anaerobic blood cultures for pediatric patients. J Pediatr. 1995;**127**:263-268. PMID: 7636652

[42] Shoji K, Komuro H, Watanabe Y, Miyairi I. The utility of anaerobic blood culture in detecting facultative anaerobic bacteremia in children. Diagn Microbiol Infect Dis. 2013;**76**:409-412. DOI: 10.1016/j.diagmicrobio.2013.05.003

[43] Brent AJ, Lakhanpaul M, Thompson M, Collier J, Ray S, Ninis N, et al. Risk score to stratify children with suspected serious bacterial infection: observational cohort study. Arch Dis Child. 2011;**96**:361-367. DOI: 10.1136/adc.2010.183111

[44] Craig DGN, Reid TWDJ, Martin KG, Davidson JS, Hayes PC, Simpson KJ. The systemic inflammatory response syndrome and sequential organ failure assessment scores are effective triage markers following paracetamol (acetaminophen) overdose. Aliment Pharmacol Ther. 2011;**34**:219-228. DOI: 10.1111/j.1365-2036.2011.04687.x

[45] Ek T, Jarfelt M, Mellander L, Abrahamsson J. Proinflammatory cytokines mediate the systemic inflammatory response associated with high-dose cytarabine treatment in children. Med Pediatr Oncol. 2001;**37**:459-464. PMID: 11745875

[46] Schwartzentruber DJ. Guidelines for the safe administration of high-dose interleukin-2. J. Immunother. 2001;**24**:287-293. PMID: 11565830

[47] Cruz AT, Perry AM, Williams EA, Graf JM, Wuestner ER, Patel B. Implementation of goal-directed therapy for children with suspected sepsis in the emergency department. Pediatrics. 2011;**127**:e758-766. DOI: 10.1542/peds.2010-2895

[48] Brierley J, Carcillo JA, Choong K, Cornell T, Decaen A, Deymann A, et al. Clinical practice parameters for hemodynamic support of pediatric and neonatal septic shock: 2007 update from the American College of Critical Care Medicine. Crit Care Med. 2009;37:666-688. DOI: 10.1097/CCM.0b013e31819323c6

[49] Delaney AP, Dan A, McCaffrey J, Finfer S. The role of albumin as a resuscitation fluid for patients with sepsis: a systematic review and meta-analysis. Crit Care Med. 2011;39:386-391. DOI: 10.1097/CCM.0b013e3181ffe217

[50] Oliveira CF, Nogueira de Sá FR, Oliveira DSF, Gottschald AFC, Moura JDG, Shibata ARO, et al. Time- and fluid-sensitive resuscitation for hemodynamic support of children in septic shock: barriers to the implementation of the American College of Critical Care Medicine/Pediatric Advanced Life Support Guidelines in a pediatric intensive care unit in a developing world. Pediatr Emerg Care. 2008;24:810-815. DOI: 10.1097/PEC.0b013e31818e9f3a

[51] Paul R, Neuman MI, Monuteaux MC, Melendez E. Adherence to PALS sepsis guidelines and hospital length of stay. Pediatrics. 2012;130:e273-280. DOI: 10.1542/peds.2012-0094

[52] Carcillo JA, Davis AL, Zaritsky A. Role of early fluid resuscitation in pediatric septic shock. JAMA. 1991;266:1242-1245. PMID: 1870250

[53] Raimer PL, Han YY, Weber MS, Annich GM, Custer JR. A normal capillary refill time of ≤ 2 seconds is associated with superior vena cava oxygen saturations of ≥70%. J Pediatr. 2011;158:968-972. DOI: 10.1016/j.jpeds.2010.11.062

[54] De Oliveira CF, de Oliveira DSF, Gottschald AFC, Moura JDG, Costa GA, Ventura AC, et al. ACCM/PALS haemodynamic support guidelines for paediatric septic shock: an outcomes comparison with and without monitoring central venous oxygen saturation. Intensive Care Med. 2008;34:1065-1075. DOI: 10.1007/s00134-008-1085-9

[55] Ceneviva G, Paschall JA, Maffei F, Carcillo JA. Hemodynamic support in fluid-refractory pediatric septic shock. Pediatrics. 1998;102:e19. PMID: 9685464

[56] Polito A, Parisini E, Ricci Z, Picardo S, Annane D. Vasopressin for treatment of vasodilatory shock: an ESICM systematic review and meta-analysis. Intensive Care Med. 2012;38:9-19. DOI: 10.1007/s00134-011-2407-x

[57] Choong K, Bohn D, Fraser DD, Gaboury I, Hutchison JS, Joffe AR, et al. Vasopressin in pediatric vasodilatory shock: a multicenter randomized controlled trial. Am J Respir Crit Care Med. 2009;180:632-639. DOI: 10.1164/rccm.200902-0221OC

[58] Rodríguez-Núñez A, López-Herce J, Gil-Antón J, Hernández A, Rey C, RETSPED Working Group of the Spanish Society of Pediatric Intensive Care. Rescue treatment with terlipressin in children with refractory septic shock: a clinical study. Crit Care. 2006;10:R20. DOI: 10.1186/cc3984

[59] Lindsay CA, Barton P, Lawless S, Kitchen L, Zorka A, Garcia J, et al. Pharmacokinetics and pharmacodynamics of milrinone lactate in pediatric patients with septic shock. J Pediatr. 1998;**132**:329-334. PMID: 9506650

[60] Irazuzta JE, Pretzlaff RK, Rowin ME. Amrinone in pediatric refractory septic shock: an open-label pharmacodynamic study. Pediatr Crit Care Med. 2001;**2**:24-28. PMID: 12797884

[61] MacLaren G, Butt W, Best D, Donath S. Central extracorporeal membrane oxygenation for refractory pediatric septic shock. Pediatr Crit Care Med. 2011;**12**:133-136. DOI: 10.1097/PCC.0b013e3181e2a4a1

[62] Skinner SC, Iocono JA, Ballard HO, Turner MD, Ward AN, Davenport DL, et al. Improved survival in venovenous vs venoarterial extracorporeal membrane oxygenation for pediatric noncardiac sepsis patients: a study of the Extracorporeal Life Support Organization registry. J Pediatr Surg. 2012;**47**:63-67. DOI: 10.1016/j.jpedsurg.2011.10.018

[63] Chastre J, Wolff M, Fagon J-Y, Chevret S, Thomas F, Wermert D, et al. Comparison of 8 vs 15 days of antibiotic therapy for ventilator-associated pneumonia in adults: a randomized trial. JAMA. 2003;**290**:2588-2598. DOI: 10.1001/jama.290.19.2588

[64] Millar M, Zhou W, Skinner R, Pizer B, Hennessy E, Wilks M, et al. Accuracy of bacterial DNA testing for central venous catheter-associated bloodstream infection in children with cancer. Health Technol Assess. 2011;**15**:1-114. DOI: 10.3310/hta15070

[65] Lacroix J, Hébert PC, Hutchison JS, Hume HA, Tucci M, Ducruet T, et al. Transfusion strategies for patients in pediatric intensive care units. N Engl J Med. 2007;**356**:1609-1619. DOI: 10.1056/NEJMoa066240

[66] Karam O, Tucci M, Ducruet T, Hume HA, Lacroix J, Gauvin F, et al. Red blood cell transfusion thresholds in pediatric patients with sepsis. Pediatr Crit Care Med. 2011;**12**:512-518. DOI: 10.1097/PCC.0b013e3181fe344b

[67] Zimmerman JJ, Williams MD. Adjunctive corticosteroid therapy in pediatric severe sepsis: observations from the RESOLVE study. Pediatr Crit Care Med. 2011;**12**:2-8. DOI: 10.1097/PCC.0b013e3181d903f6

[68] Markovitz BP, Goodman DM, Watson RS, Bertoch D, Zimmerman J. A retrospective cohort study of prognostic factors associated with outcome in pediatric severe sepsis: what is the role of steroids? Pediatr Crit Care Med. 2005;**6**:270-274. DOI: 10.1097/01.PCC.0000160596.31238.72

[69] Randolph AG. Management of acute lung injury and acute respiratory distress syndrome in children. Crit Care Med. 2009;**37**:2448-2454. DOI: 10.1097/CCM.0b013e3181aee5dd

[70] Branco RG, Garcia PCR, Piva JP, Casartelli CH, Seibel V, Tasker RC. Glucose level and risk of mortality in pediatric septic shock. Pediatr Crit Care Med. 2005;**6**:470-472. DOI: 10.1097/01.PCC.0000161284.96739.3A

[71] Odetola FO, Gebremariam A, Freed GL. Patient and hospital correlates of clinical outcomes and resource utilization in severe pediatric sepsis. Pediatrics. 2007;**119**:487-494. DOI: 10.1542/peds.2006-2353

[72] Watson RS, Carcillo JA, Linde-Zwirble WT, Clermont G, Lidicker J, Angus DC. The epidemiology of severe sepsis in children in the United States. Am J Respir Crit Care Med. 2003;**167**:695-701. DOI: 10.1164/rccm.200207-682OC

[73] Han YY, Carcillo JA, Dragotta MA, Bills DM, Watson RS, Westerman ME, et al. Early reversal of pediatric-neonatal septic shock by community physicians is associated with improved outcome. Pediatrics. 2003;**112**:793-799. PMID: 14523168

[74] Czaja AS, Zimmerman JJ, Nathens AB. Readmission and late mortality after pediatric severe sepsis. Pediatrics. 2009;**123**:849-857. DOI: 10.1542/peds.2008-0856

[75] Van de Voorde P, Emerson B, Gomez B, Willems J, Yildizdas D, Iglowstein I, et al. Paediatric community-acquired septic shock: results from the REPEM network study. Eur J Pediatr. 2013;**172**:667-674. DOI: 10.1007/s00431-013-1930-x

Infections and Multidrug-Resistant Pathogens in ICU Patients

Muntean Delia and Licker Monica

Abstract

This chapter aims to highlight the main types of infections in the ICU, in order to improve diagnostic and therapeutic management. Risk factors for patients hospitalised in the ICU will be raised: the increasing use of invasive devices and procedures, aggressive antimicrobial therapies, surgical interventions, immunosuppressive treatments or co-morbidities responsible for immune deficiencies. Starting from the rising mortality risk among patients with hospital-acquired infections (HAI), in the case of failure to control the pathogen in the first 24–48 h, we will tackle about the prevention, reduction and control of the emergence of resistant pathogens. The rational administration of antibiotics will also be addressed, with the aim of reducing adverse reactions, including secondary infections, decreasing the mortality rate, length of hospital stay and costs of health care.

Keywords: ventilator-associated pneumonia, intra-vascular catheter-related bacteraemia, sever sepsis, septic shock, antimicrobial treatment, multidrug resistance

1. Introduction

Modern medicine is a tributary to a continuously increasing degree of diagnostic and therapeutic invasiveness. In particular, intensive care units (ICUs) are confronted with increasing number of patients with marked co-morbidities, severe acute pathology or immune suppression, and intrinsic infectious risk factors. Additionally, given the pathogenicity changes of potentially hospital-acquired pathogens, most healthcare-associated infections (HCAIs) are caused by multidrug-resistant organisms (MDRO).

2. ICU infections

2.1. Severe respiratory infections

Pneumonia is one of the infections frequently requiring hospital admission and urgent antimicrobial treatment due to the risk of rapid evolution to respiratory and multiple organ failure, especially in immunocompromised patients, or when caused by MDRO. The diagnosis of severe pneumonia requires ICU admission given the need for assisted ventilation or oxygen therapy, in the presence of radiological changes, confirming the rapid progression, as well as the evolution towards sepsis [1, 2].

Community-acquired pneumonia (CAP) is caused by bacteria in 85% of cases, the most frequently involved pathogens being *Streptococcus pneumoniae, Haemophilus influenzae* and *Moraxella catarrhalis*. Severe CAP cases may also be produced by other pathogens (influenza viruses, coronaviruses, Hanta virus, *Legionella*).

Pneumonia may trigger acute myocardial infarction in patients with heart diseases, while in splenectomised patients or with spleen dysfunction, *S. pneumoniae* may cause severe sepsis with lethal outcome within 12–24 h from onset, even under antibiotic therapy.

The treatment of CAP must cover both typical and atypical pathogens. Clinical studies have shown that monotherapy with respiratory fluoroquinolones or tigecycline is almost as effective as therapy with antibiotic associations (ceftriaxone plus doxycycline, azithromycin, or respiratory quinolones) [3].

On the other hand, presently ICUs are especially confronted with respiratory infections acquired during hospitalisation. According to 2012/506/EU European Parliament Decision, hospital-acquired pneumonia (HAP) occurs 48 h or more after admission and was not incubating at the time of admission, while ventilated-associated pneumonia (VAP) arises in 48 h after endotracheal intubation [4]. The microorganisms involved in the aetiology of these pneumonia cases originate in the oropharyngeal or upper airways colonisation flora or by direct inoculation of contaminated solutions, via an endotracheal catheter, or exogenous contamination of respiratory equipment caused by health care staff.

The hospital-acquired risk factors associated with this type of infection are:

- long time sedation,
- general anaesthesia with endotracheal intubation,
- other invasive procedures: bronchoscopy, nasogastric catheterisation,
- prolonged use of assisted ventilation,
- reintubation, change of ventilation circuits at intervals under 48 h,
- post-trauma intubation,
- tracheostomy,
- corticotherapy or other immunosuppressive treatments,

- antibiotic therapy, administration of antacids or H_2 blockers, barbituric therapy after cranial traumas,

- thoracic or upper abdominal surgery,

- emergency surgery,

- administration of over 4 units of blood before the surgical intervention [5, 6].

These factors disturb respiratory functions leading to obstructions, decreased pulmonary volume, decreased filtration of inhaled air, and decreased secretion clearance. The insertion of an endotracheal tube allows the direct access of pathogens into the lower airways or may cause lesions of the epithelial mucosa, which represent breaches. Additionally, inadequate hand hygiene of medical personnel, lack of adherence to universal precautions, errors in decontamination of equipment or in the practice of endotracheal aspiration may favour not only cross-contamination but also the direct access of a massive bacterial inoculum.

This pneumonia is caused by a wide range of pathogens, and it may be plurietiological and is only rarely caused by viruses or fungi. The aetiological agents frequently involved in such infections are not only Gram-negative bacilli (*Pseudomonas aeruginosa*, *Klebsiella* spp., *Escherichia coli*) but also Gram-positive cocci such as *Staphylococcus aureus*. The frequency of MDRO is increasing and influences the treatment, as in the case of methicillin-resistant *Staphylococcus aureus* (MRSA), carbapenem-resistant *Pseudomonas*, fluoroquinolones, antipseudomonal penicillins and cephalosporins, extended-spectrum beta-lactamase-producing *Enterobacteriaceae* (ESBL), *Acinetobacter baumannii*, etc. The risk factors for MDRO infections are the use of antibiotics during the previous 90 days, the onset of pneumonia after 4 days of hospitalisation, circulation of such pathogens in the health care unit in question, as well as the presence of comorbidities (immune suppression or immunosuppressive treatments).

The diagnosis of HAP should be rapidly reached, and the antibiotic treatment has to be promptly introduced, and any delay potentially aggravates the evolution and prognosis. The first antibiotic of choice depends on infection severity, patient's risk factors, and the number of hospitalisation days accumulated until the onset of pneumonia.

The empirical treatment of HAP or VAP occurring during the first five hospitalisation days in patients without risk factors for MDRO must include antibiotics active against not only aerobic Gram-negative bacilli (*Enterobacter* spp., *E. coli*, *Klebsiella* spp., *Proteus* spp., *Serratia* spp.), pathogens with respiratory tropism (*Haemophilus influenzae* and *Streptococcus pneumoniae*), but also methicillin-sensitive *S. aureus* (MSSA). Recommendations include therapeutic schemes based on ceftriaxone or a fluoroquinolone (ciprofloxacin or levofloxacin) or ampicillin-sulbactam or ertapenem (**Figure 1**).

In the case of patients with HAP or VAP who are at risk for MDRO infection, regardless of the infection's severity, the antibiotic treatment must be directed against *P. aeruginosa*, *K. pneumoniae* (ESBL-producing strains), *Acinetobacter* spp. and MRSA. Antibiotic associations including antipseudomonal cephalosporins (ceftazidime), an antipseudomonal carbapenem (imipenem) or beta-lactam/beta-lactamase inhibitors (piperacillin-tazobactam), will be administered, in association with antipseudomonal fluoroquinolones (ciprofloxacin) or an

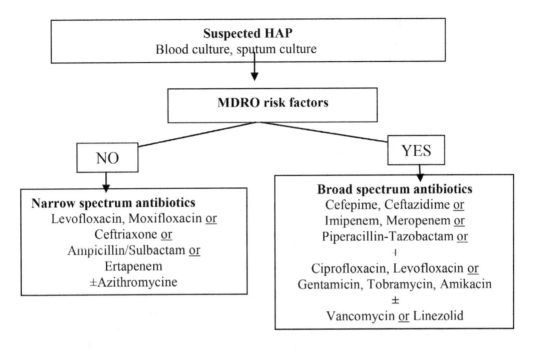

Figure 1. Antibiotic therapy in HAP.

Antibiotic	Adult Doses
Broad-spectrum cephalosporins	
Cefepime	1-2 g every 8-12 hours
Ceftazidime	2 g every 8 hours
Carbapenems	
Imipenem	500 mg every 6 hours or 1 g every 8 hours
Meropenem	1 g every 8 hours
Betalactam/ beta-lactamase inhibitor	
Piperacillin-tazobactam	4.5 g every 6 hours
Aminoglycosides	
Gentamicin	7 mg/kg/day
Tobramycin	7 mg/kg/day
Amikacin	20 mg/kg/day
Fluoroquinolones	
Levofloxacin	750 mg/day
Ciprofloxacin	400 mg every 8 hours
Anti-MRSA antibiotics	
Vancomycin	15 mg/kg every 12 hours
Linezolid	600 mg every 12 hours

Table 1. Empirical antibiotic treatment of HAP with MDRO.

aminoglycoside (tobramycin) and vancomycin or linezolid, to cover MRSA. If a *Legionella* infection is suspected, a macrolide (azithromycin) must also be associated [7] (**Table 1**).

The duration of the antibiotic treatment in HAP must be adjusted to the severity of the disease, the time required to obtain clinical improvement and the aetiological agent, but it has to exceed with at least 3 days the time to clinical improvement. The clinical response occurs after at least 48–72 h, a period during which the recommendation is to maintain the therapeutic scheme. If, after this interval of empirical treatment, the clinical status of the patient did not improve, the therapeutic scheme must be broadened, potential complications (pleurisy, pulmonary abscess) and/or non-infectious causes must be sought.

2.2. Bacteraemia and septicaemia

2.2.1. Generalised septicaemic infections

The generalised septicaemic infection is an infection with an unpredictable outcome, high severity and increased mortality in the absence of adequate treatment. The correct choice of empirical antibiotic treatment depends on the intelligent use of clinical knowledge and epidemiological and microbiological data regarding the pathology in the area where the patient comes from. The lack of knowledge on the local resistance prevalence is a predictive factor for an incorrect treatment. The basic principle, which guides the treatment of the critical patient, is to rapidly initiate antibiotic treatment at correct doses, concordant with the pharmacokinetic and pharmacodynamic characters of the chosen drug and to adapt the treatment to the changes occurring in the clinical evolution and to the results of the antimicrobial sensitivity tests as soon as these become available.

Immediately after a patient with suspected sepsis is admitted, an attentive anamnesis and a thorough clinical examination are conducted in order to establish the entry and the location of the primary and secondary septic sites. The first emergency microbiological investigations are conducted (repeated blood cultures, cultures from secretions, lesions, urine, sputum, exudates, pleural fluid, etc.) together with evaluations of the renal, hepatic functions and state of consciousness, thus determining the severity of the case [8, 9].

The practical approach includes the emergency admission of the patient into the ICU where prevention or correction of hypovolemia, functional and metabolic dysfunctions are attempted, concomitantly with the prompt initiation of antibiotic treatment according to the maximal probability criterion.

The correct antibiotic treatment targets the resident microbial flora in the organ presumed to be the source of the infectious process.

The empirical treatment of sepsis consists of the association of bactericidal antibiotics with synergistic actions or monotherapy with an ultra-broad-spectrum antibiotic; antibiotics are administered intravenously in order to rapidly achieve an effective concentration in the infection site.

Empirical antibiotic therapy proved to be equally effective in beta-lactam-aminoglycoside associations, monotherapy with carbapenems, broad-spectrum penicillins/beta-lactamase inhibitors (ticarcillin/clavulanic acid, piperacillin/tazobactam) or third- and fourth-generation cephalosporins [10].

The aetiology of sepsis varies with the age of the patient, and the empirical treatment must be adapted to the most probable aetiology, but correlated with age, weight and associated pathology.

Adults with severe sepsis of unknown source must be treated with antibiotics effective against Gram-negative bacilli, *Staphylococcus aureus*, streptococci, respectively carbapenems (meropenem or imipenem) plus vancomycin. Septic shock requires the urgent refilling of the vascular system by infusions with saline solutions until the central venous pressure is re-established (over 80 mm at 6 h from hospital admission); at the same time, the primary source of infection is investigated, blood culture is collected and the first dose of antibiotic is administered, knowing that the time from admission to the initiation of antibiotic therapy is the strongest prognostic factor.

Patients admitted in a state of septic or toxic-septic shock will not be treated with beta-lactam (The bacterial load is very high, the pathogens are in a stationary phase with low protein synthesis, hence with a low synthesis of penicillin-binding proteins, so antibiotics lack their target.)

Colistin has a rapid antibacterial effect completed by a significant post-antibiotic effect against *P. aeruginosa*, *A. baumannii* and *K. pneumoniae*. The most effective administration regimen is at 8 h. Colistin proved an important alternative in the treatment of MDR Gram-negative bacilli. Resistance to colistin is caused by sub-optimal doses. Colistin dosage must be optimised, as this antibiotic is the last option in the treatment of MDRO [11–13].

When a biliary infection is suspected to be at the origin of bacteraemia, the most frequently encountered bacteria are enterococci and aerobic Gram-negative bacilli, which respond well to piperacillin/tazobactam or ticarcillin/clavulanate; alternatively, ceftriaxone, ciprofloxacin or levofloxacin associated to metronidazole may be administered.

A great part (around 25%) of sepsis cases occur as a result of community or hospital-acquired urinary tract infections (UTI), evolving with a renal or complication of prostatic parenchyma. In such cases, the time from hospital admission to the initiation of antibiotic treatment is also decisive for the evolution. After collection of samples for blood and urine cultures, the first dose of broad-spectrum antibiotic active against *E.coli*, *Proteus* spp., *Enterobacter* spp., *Klebsiella* spp., *P. aeruginosa* is administered; more rare cases of sepsis of urinary origin may be caused by Gram-positive bacteria (15%) or by *Pseudomonas* spp., especially in patients with immune deficits. For an effective treatment of community-acquired urosepsis, depending on the type of local susceptibility, a third-generation cephalosporin or a fluoroquinolone may be indicated; in urosepsis following urologic surgery in patients with long-term urinary catheters, the association of a third-generation cephalosporin active against *Pseudomonas* or piperacillin/tazobactam with an aminoglycoside or a carbapenem is useful, this association being required to cover MDRO [14].

It should be noted that treatment in sepsis is complex, antibiotic therapy being accompanied with measures to eradicate the entry site and septic metastases, to correct tissue hypoxia and to maintain hydro-electrolyte and acid-base balance.

2.2.2. Infections associated with invasive devices

Invasive devices (endotracheal, intra-vascular catheters) increase the risk of HCAI especially with MDRO, by colonisation and biofilm formation on the internal surface of these devices. All types of intra-vascular devices may become complicated with blood infections, but arterial catheters used for the haemodynamic monitoring and peripheral catheters show lower infection risks than central venous caterers (**Table 2**).

The removal of intra-vascular, gastric or bladder catheters, neurosurgical shunts, etc. as soon as they are no longer needed, represents an infection prevention measure. Both their insertion and removal is done by specialised staff, trained to work under sterile conditions, avoiding the risk of contamination. Knowing that invasive devices, catheters included, are the most frequent cause of HCAIs, their insertion must be conducted under aseptic conditions, choosing the most suitable site (for instance, sub-clavian rather than femoral), after ensuring the asepsis of the cutaneous area, preferably with chlorhexidine, and not with alcohol or iodine solutions. In severely immunocompromised patients, the recommendation is to use antibiotic-impregnated catheters. Clinical studies confirm the significant reduction in catheter-associated infections when these are removed as soon as their role is no longer essential [15–17].

An increasing number of patients require central venous catheters for long periods of time (for haemodialysis, total parenteral nutrition, chemotherapy), which favours complications such as thrombosis or infection. Central venous catheter-associated bacteraemia imposes the removal of the catheter and systemic administration of antibiotics. The clinical decision to remove a catheter suspected of infection relies on the presence of local infection signs. The decision to maintain the device is made in the absence of severity signs in patients with technical difficulties of catheter reinsertion in a new site.

There are situations when catheters may not be removed or replaced (lack of venous approach, counter indication of a new intervention, etc.). In such cases, attempts are made to save the venous line by eliminating the intra-luminal colonisation before the onset of bacteraemia or, once bacteraemia is present, the general administration of antibiotic is associated with exposing the inner surface of the catheter, after its closure, at a very high concentration of the adequate antibiotic meant to eradicate the colonisation. This technique proved effective in the case of Gram-negative bacilli and coagulase-negative staphylococci, but it is not recommended in colonisations with *S. aureus* [18].

2.3. Urinary tract infections

UTIs are the most frequent HCAIs. In most hospitals, catheter-related bacteriuria represents 40% of all HCAI within 1 year. The decision to treat is made after discriminating between the presence of bacteria (colonisation) and symptomatic infectious processes. The signs of

Risk factors	Risk distribution
Type of catheter	Polyvinylchloride > teflon > polyurethane, metallic
Catheter site	Central > peripheral
	Femoral > jugular > subclavian
	Lower limbs > upper limbs
Type of placement	By incision > percutaneous
Duration of placement	over 72h > under 72h
Manner of placement	In emergency > selective
Experience of medical staff	Unexperienced staff > specially trained teams

Table 2. Distribution of the infection risk in the intra-vascular catheterisation.

catheter-associated UTIs are fever, lateral lumbar pain, sensitivity in the costovertebral angle, haematuria and delirium with recent onset. After catheter removal, pollakiuria or dysuria may be present.

The Infectious Disease Society of America defines asymptomatic bacteriuria as the absence of symptoms with the presence of over 10^5 colony forming units/ml of one or more bacterial species in a catheterised patient. In most cases of asymptomatic bacteriuria, the treatment led to the temporary sterilisation of urine and not to the eradication of pathogens [19]. Additionally, in 33–50% of patients, after catheter removal, the bacteriuria spontaneously resolved. This is why treating an asymptomatic bacteriuria increases the risk of antimicrobial resistance or of adverse reactions associated with useless antibiotic treatment.

Some pathogenic bacteria produce biofilms, which consist of an adherent layer of microorganisms and their extracellular products. The biofilm protects the pathogens against the host's defence mechanisms and against antibiotic therapy. Migration to the urinary bladder occurs in 1–3 days. The duration of catheterization is an important risk factor, with almost all patients who are catheterised for more than 30 days developing bacteriuria. These patients are at risk of upper urinary tract inflammation, which increases the risk of bacteraemia. Infections linked to long-term catheterisation are often polymicrobial, which involves a broad-spectrum treatment.

The selection of antibiotics used for the treatment of catheter-associated UTIs depends on the result of the microscopical examination, as well as on the colonial characters. In 60–80% of cases, the causative agent is a Gram-negative bacillus (*E.coli*, *Klebsiella* spp., *Pseudomonas* spp., *Proteus* spp., *Enterobacter* spp.). The remaining 20–40% is caused by Gram-positive bacteria, most often species of staphylococci or enterococci. The empirical treatment has to take the following factors, which increase the risk of antibiotic resistance: the duration of hospitalisation, previous administration of antibiotics, and local resistance patterns.

Urinary fluoroquinolones (ciprofloxacin and levofloxacin) are administered to patients with mild and moderate infections, who are considered haemodynamically stable and do not present an altered mental status. Moxifloxacin is not recommended, as it does not reach effective urine concentrations. Broad-spectrum cephalosporins, ceftriaxone or cefepime, may also be used. In patients with urosepsis or in those haemodynamically unstable (hypothermia, tachycardia over 90/minute, tachypnoea over 20 respirations/minute or Pco_2 under 33 mmHg, leukocytosis over 12,000/mm^3 or leukopenia under 4000/mm^3) piperacillin-tazobactam is administered.

In medium clinical forms, ciprofloxacin, 400 mg iv, for every 12 h or levofloxacin 500 mg iv /24 h or ceftriaxone for 1 g iv/day are administered.

The recommended treatments in severe forms include: cefepime 2 g iv/12 h, ceftazidime 2 g iv/8 h, imipenem 500 mg iv/6 h, doripenem 500 mg iv/8 h, meropenem 1 g/8 h and piperacillin/tazobactam 3.375 g iv/6 h.

The treatment of UTIs associated with bladder catheterisation is done with antibiotics for 3 days in women aged over 65 years, from whom the catheter has been removed; otherwise, the treatment is given for 7 days. The duration of levofloxacin treatment is 5 days.

Most hospital-acquired UTIS are expensive and may be prevented. The implementation of protocols based on present guidelines will reduce the inadequate use, as well as the antimicrobial resistance. When catheterisation is necessary, its duration should be limited. In case infections occur, the empirical treatment should be conducted according to the suspected pathogens and on the hospital's antibiogram. When the results of cultures become available, antibiotics narrow their spectrum. The treatment should be limited to 7–14 days, depending on the response to treatment. Catheter removal is a key factor because catheterisation increases the risk for hospital-acquired UTI and other complications, resulting in prolonged hospitalisation and increased costs [20, 21].

2.4. Intra-abdominal infections

Intra-abdominal infections include a series of diseases with variable severity, from uncomplicated appendicitis to faecal peritonitis. Uncomplicated infections involve a single organ and may not reach the peritoneum, and they may be solved either by surgical resection or by administration of antibiotics. Complicated intra-abdominal infections are those which extend to the peritoneum causing localised or generalised peritonitis; in order to solve these, the infection source must be solved by both surgery and antibiotic therapy.

The antimicrobial therapy of intra-abdominal infections, which are to be solved percutaneously or by surgery, has the following goals: to accelerate the elimination of the infecting microorganisms, to decrease the recurrence risk of the intra-abdominal infection, to shorten the clinical evolution, to limit the expansion of the infection to the abdominal wall and to decrease the risk of generalisation of the infectious process.

The antibiotic therapy is initiated after hydroelectrolyte rebalance, the restored volemia determining the restoration of the visceral perfusion and a better distribution of the medication. Moreover, this diminishes the side effects of antibiotics, which have been exacerbated by the deficitary perfusion of internal organs.

The empirical antibiotic treatment is initiated in concordance with the most probable microbiological spectrum, the type and density of germs being dependant on the level where the perforation of the digestive tract has occurred. By gastric, duodenal and proximal jejunal perforations, a low number of aerobic Gram-positive and anaerobic Gram-negative bacteria, generally sensitive to cephalosporins, are released into the peritoneum. *Candida albicans* has also been isolated, but antifungal treatment is only required in the case of patients under immunosuppressive treatment or in patients with recurrent intra-abdominal infections. The perforations of the distal small intestine often evolve as localised abscesses and peritonitis only takes place when these are ruptured. The intra-abdominal infections propagated from the colon into the peritoneum are caused by anaerobic or facultative anaerobic Gram-negative bacteria; *Bacteroides fragilis* is sometimes present.

The selection of the antibiotic should then be guided by the results of the cultures from the biological specimens obtained by percutaneous drainage or during the surgical intervention, but until these become available, it is necessary and useful to perform the microscopical examination directly on a Gram-stained smear. If high numbers of Gram-positive cocci are present, these are very likely to be enterococci or other faecal streptococci, which imposes the association of vancomycin.

Aerobic and anaerobic Gram-negative cocci may be covered by administration of cefoxitin, ampicillin/sulbactam, piperacillin/tazobactam, imipenem, meropenem, moxifloxacin, while aerobic Gram-negative bacilli may be destroyed with aminoglycosides, second-, third- and fourth-generation cephalosporins, aztreonam, antipseudomonal penicillins or fluoroquinolones (ciprofloxacin, levofloxacin). It must be mentioned that ertapenem is not active on *Pseudomonas aeruginosa* and *Acinetobacter* spp., and in the case of critical patients infected with *P. aeruginosa*, the dose of meropenem must be increased to 1 g administered for every 6 h. Vancomycin-resistant enterococci produce extremely difficult to treat infections, the only useful antibiotic being daptomycin. Tigecycline has been approved for the treatment of complicated intra-abdominal infections caused by *Citrobacter freundii*, *Enterobacter cloacae*, *E. coli*, *Klebsiella oxytoca*, *Klebsiella pneumoniae*, *Enterococcus faecalis* (vancomycin-susceptible), MSSA, MRSA and some anaerobic bacteria [22].

The antibiotic, which is active only against Gram-negative bacilli and anaerobic bacteria, is metronidazole, for which no resistance has been reported.

The patients at high risk of unfavourable evolution and reserved prognosis have a high APACHE II score, poor nutritional status, significant cardiovascular diseases, immune suppression induced by medicines or by co-morbidities, while the infection source cannot be controlled. The predictive factors of therapeutic failure include the duration of the evolution prior to hospital admission, more than 2 days of presurgical treatment, as well as the presence of the MDRO. These patients should be treated similarly to those with hospital-acquired infections with carbapenems and vancomycin, but also considering the local antibiotic resistance.

The antibiotic treatment must be administered until the resolution of the clinical signs of infection (normalisation of the thermal curve, restoration of the intestinal transit) and normalisation of the biological inflammatory syndrome.

In cases with recurrent intra-abdominal infections, the diagnosis must be reassessed after 5–7 days of treatment and the investigations should be broadened (echography, CT). Often, the antibiotic therapy must be adjusted or a new surgical intervention is required in order to eliminate the site of infection.

2.5. Meningitis

The antibiotic treatment must be urgently initiated, immediately after blood collection for blood culture and after performing the lumbar puncture. Delayed administration of the first dose of antibiotic is associated with an aggravated prognosis, and it is a strong independent factor of increased mortality, exceeding the importance of disease severity upon hospital admission and of the isolation of a penicillin-resistant strain.

The most frequent cause of delayed antibiotic therapy is the missed diagnosis due to an atypical form of meningitis (absence of fever, headache or neck stiffness). Another possible cause of temporization is represented by scheduling the imagistic investigation immediately after admitting the patient in whom the spinal tap is not safe: risk of a cerebral hernia after cerebrospinal fluid (CSF) collection, in cases of expansive intra-cranial processes accompanied by papilledema or focal signs. In this latter situation, computerised tomography (CT) or nuclear magnetic resonance (NMR) examinations should be conducted after blood collection for blood culture and after the first dose of antibiotic, despite the risk of excessive treatment.

The antibiotic administration route in meningitis is intravenous, which is capable to ensure the CSF bactericidal concentrations; the exception is for rifampicin, which may be administered orally and is useful in the treatment of meningitis caused by beta-lactam-resistant pneumococcus and coagulase-negative staphylococci.

Antibiotic selection: in the treatment of bacterial meningitis, bactericidal antibiotics able to cross the blood-brain barrier are administered, so that optimal CSF concentrations are ensured regardless of the meningeal inflammation degree (meningeal inflammation favours the penetration of the antibiotic in the sub-arachnoid space at the onset of the disease, but as the inflammation regresses under treatment, the concentration tends to decrease, so that higher doses are required as compared to other diseases) [23].

Patients with suspected bacterial meningitis will be initially treated with a broad-spectrum antibiotic concordant to the most probable aetiology, the selection being made depending on the age and comorbidities. After establishing the aetiology and antibiotic susceptibility of the isolated pathogen, the antibiotic therapy will be focused, maintaining the high doses and intravenous administration.

The lumbar puncture should be repeated after the first 24–36 h from the initiation of the treatment in order to assess CSF cytological, biochemical and bacteriological changes.

The immune competent adult with bacterial meningitis requires an initial antibiotic treatment aiming at meningococcus and pneumococcus, consisting in the association of ceftriaxone (2 g/12 h) or cefotaxime (2 g/6 h) with vancomycin (30–60 mg/kg/day for every 8 or 12 h); third-generation cephalosporins must be administered even if the antibiogram shows that the respective strain presents intermediate sensitivity or resistance, because vancomycin acts synergically and increases the efficiency of the therapy [24].

Patients with bacterial meningitis and compromised cell immunity due to pre-existing conditions or immunosuppressive treatment, but with conserved renal function, should be treated with vancomycin (60 mg/kg/day divided into two or three doses) plus cefepime (6 g/day divided into three doses) or meropenem (6 g/day divided into three doses).

If a *Listeria* infection is suspected, the empirical treatment may consist in the association between vancomycin and moxifloxacin (400 mg in a single daily dose) plus trimethoprim-sulfamethoxazole (10–20 mg/kg/day divided at 6 or 12 h).

The duration of the antibiotic treatment in meningitis is not standardised, but it should be individualised based upon the clinical response of each patient, but usually 7 days of treatment is sufficient for meningococcal and *H. influenzae* meningitis, 10–14 days for pneumococcal meningitis, 14–21 days for meningitis with *S. agalactiae* and 21 days or more for meningitis with *L. monocytogenes*; meningitis with aerobic Gram-negative bacilli requires antibiotic administration for 21 or 14 days after the last CSF sterile culture.

Hospital-acquired bacterial meningitis (HABM) may be the result of an invasive procedure (craniotomy, insertion of internal or external ventricular catheter, lumbar puncture, intrathecal medication, spinal anaesthesia), of a complicated cranial trauma or, in more rare cases, of an infectious metastasis in patients with hospital-acquired bacteraemia. Such meningitis is caused by microorganisms with different spectra from community-acquired cases, and the disease is the result of particular pathogenetic mechanisms.

Bacterial meningitis is a redoubtable complication of craniotomy, occurring in 0.8–1.5% of the patients who undergo this procedure. One-third of the post-craniotomy meningitis cases develop during the first week after the surgical intervention, another third during the second week and one-third after the second week from the intervention, sometimes even years after the surgical procedure. The risk of post-surgical meningitis may be minimised by the attentive use of surgical techniques, especially those which decrease the possibility of liquid fistulae. Other factors associated with meningitis after craniotomy include concomitant infection at the incision site and duration of procedure exceeding 4 h.

The incidence of meningitis associated with internal ventricular catheters (cerebrospinal shunt) used in the treatment of hydrocephaly varies between 4 and 17%. The most important causative factor is the colonisation of the catheter at the time of insertion so that most infections become manifest in less than 1 month from the procedure.

External ventricular catheters are used to monitor intra-cranial pressure or to temporarily deviate the CSF if there is an obstruction in the system or as a treatment component in cases of infection of the internal catheter. The rate of external catheter-associated infection is around 8%.

The incidence of meningitis after moderate or severe cranial trauma is 1.4%. The open cranial trauma is encountered in 5% of cranial trauma and is complicated by meningitis in 2–11% of cases. Most patients in whom meningitis occurs as a complication of closed cranial trauma present a skull base fracture, which creates a communication between the sub-arachnoid space and the sinus cavities, posing an infection risk of up to 25%. The average time interval between the trauma and the onset of meningitis is 11 days. The CSF leak is the major risk factor, even though most post-traumatic leaks are not diagnosed. Most fistulae resolve spontaneously within 7 days, a surgical intervention is recommended if the breach persists. The cranial trauma is the most frequent cause of recurrent meningitis.

The diagnostic procedure relies on neuroimagistic investigations, CSF analysis (cell count, biochemical tests for glucose, proteins, Gram staining, cultures) and blood cultures. Neuroimagistics is indicated in most patients as it allows the ventricular size evaluation and brings information on a possible poor functioning of the shunt or the presence of residual catheters after previous surgical interventions.

The most frequently encountered bacteria in these cases are Gram-negative bacilli (*Klebsiella pneumoniae, Pseudomonas aeruginosa*), *S. aureus* and coagulase-negative staphylococci.

The empirical antibiotic therapy in HABM depends on the pathogenesis of the infectious process. In patients with meningitis occurring after neurosurgical interventions, or in patients with long-term hospitalisation after open cranial trauma or skull base fractures, vancomycin is associated with cefepime, ceftazidime or meropenem; the second antibiotic is selected depending on the local chemotherapeutics susceptibility profiles of Gram-negative bacilli. The empirical treatment in skull base fracture or early after ENT surgery includes vancomycin plus a third-generation cephalosporin (cefotaxime, ceftriaxone). After isolating the involved pathogen, antimicrobial therapy is changed for an optimal management. Linezolid and daptomycin are effective in staphylococcal meningitis; linezolid has good pharmacokinetic properties—CSF penetration is around 80%.

The initiation of empirical treatment is recommended in all patients with post-surgical signs of meningitis; this is withdrawn after 72 h in case the results of CSF cultures are negative. The treatment must be individualised, especially in patients previously treated with antibiotics, in whom the treatment is continued despite the negative results of cultures.

Given the emergence of MDR Gram-negative bacilli, the antimicrobial therapy of HABM caused by these pathogens becomes problematic. This is especially true in cases of HABM caused by *Acinetobacter baumannii* species, bacteria with acquired resistance to third- and fourth-generation cephalosporins and even to carbapenems. The treatment of *Acinetobacter* meningitis includes meropenem associated with an aminoglycoside administered intra-ventricularly or intrathecally. If the identified isolate is resistant to carbapenems, intra-ventricular or intrathecal administration of colistin or polymyxin B will be given instead of meropenem.

Treatment protocols recommended depending on the pathogenesis of the infectious process:

- *Infection after neurosurgical procedure*—Gram-negative bacilli (including *P. aeruginosa*), *Staphylococcus aureus* and coagulase-negative staphylococci (*S. epidermidis*) may be involved. Vancomycin plus cefepime or meropenem are recommended.

- *Ventricular or lumbar catheter*—coagulase-negative staphylococci, *S. aureus*, Gram-negative bacilli (*P. aeruginosa*) and *Propionibacterium acnes* may be present. Vancomycin plus cefepime or meropenem are recommended.

- *Penetrating trauma*: *S. aureus*, coagulase-negative staphylococci, Gram-negative bacilli. Vancomycin plus cefepime or meropenem is administered.

- *Skull base fracture*: Streptococcus pneumoniae, Haemophilus influenzae, Streptococcus pyogenes. Vancomycin plus a third-generation cephalosporin (ceftriaxone or cefotaxime) is recommended.

2.6. Infections of the skin and soft tissues

With the increasing incidence of MRSA, skin and soft tissue infections require more frequent admission of patients presenting tissue necrosis, fever, hypotension, intense pain, altered consciousness, respiratory, hepatic or renal failure, to the ICU. When choosing the therapeutic scheme, the possibility of a polymicrobial infection must be considered, with consecutive need to cover not only MRSA but also Gram-negative and anaerobic bacteria. An inadequate initial empirical treatment is associated with prolonged evolution and hospital stay [25].

Perianal infections and abscesses, infected decubitus ulcers, and moderate and severe infections of the diabetic foot frequently involve multiple aetiologies and require coverage for streptococci, MRSA, aerobic and anaerobic Gram-negative bacilli until the results of microbiological investigations become available.

In the case of patients with non-suppurative cellulitis, a beta-lactam antibiotic, such as cefazolin, may be initially prescribed, which is to be replaced in case of unsatisfactory clinical evolution. The replacement will be made according to the result of the antimicrobial susceptibility test or with an antibiotic active on MRSA, if the pathogen has not been isolated in the culture. The empirical treatment of MRSA infections may include vancomycin, linezolid, daptomycin, tigecycline and telavancin. Linezolid, daptomycin, vancomycin and telavancin additionally also cover streptococcal infections and not only MRSA.

In case of a documented or suspected staphylococcal infection, the recommendation is to immediately initiate the antibiotic treatment according to maximal probability criteria and according to local data on the sensitivity of strains circulating in the respective area. The doses of antibiotic must be adequate, because sub-inhibitory concentrations favour the release of staphylococcal toxins and virulence factors (PVL—Panton-Valentine leukocidin), which trigger the onset of skin, lung or bone necrotic lesions. Catheters and intra-vascular devices must be removed. In cases with detected abscesses, these should be drained; the localised infection of a prosthetic joint requires the removal of the prosthesis, but if the infection is located on a valvular prosthesis, its removal is not always required.

The treatment of MRSA infections frequently includes the administration of vancomycin. The increased vancomycin consumption has posed an increasing selection pressure of staphylococcal strains resistant to this antibiotic. The concentration of vancomycin required to inhibit most *S. aureus* strains is 0.5–2 mg/l. The strains with a minimum inhibitory concentration (MIC) of vancomycin between 8 and 16 mg/l are classified as intermediate sensitive or VISA (vancomycin-intermediate *S. aureus*), while strains with MIC ≥32 mg/l are considered resistant or vancomycin-resistant *S. aureus* (VRSA). The resistance mechanisms are different in the two types of strains: in VISA strains, the bacterial cell wall is thickened by the altered biosynthesis process and the glycopeptides targets are hidden in its thickness and in the case of VRSA strains, the target of glycopeptides is itself modified.

Surgical wound infections are another category of infections frequently confronting ICUs. In their most frequently polymicrobial aetiology, Gram-positive cocci (especially MRSA), *Enterobacteriaceae* and non-fermentative Gram-negative bacilli (*P. aeruginosa*) are among the most frequently isolated pathogens. The empirical treatment of these infections consists of associating cefepime or meropenem with an aminoglycoside or a fluoroquinolone.

Many extrinsic risk factors are inter-connected with intrinsic factors or are found in association, for which reason, the Study on the Efficacy of Nosocomial Infections Control (SENIC), a risk index, has been proposed for surgical wound infections. When compared to the traditional Altemeier system, this index predicts the risk of post-surgical infection two times better and the inclusion of other items does not seem to improve its predictive capacity [26]. The National Surveillance System of Nosocomial Infections in the USA proposed the NNIS risk index, further completed with the item on the use of laparoscopic techniques (**Tables 3** and **4**).

SENIC index		NNIS index	
Item	Score	Item	
1. Operating time > 2 ore	1 point	1. Class ASA 3/ 4/ 5	1 point
2. Abdominal surgery	1 point	2. Contaminated or septic surgery	1 point
3. Contaminated or septic surgery	1 point	3. Duration of surgical procedure > T (variable time depending on the operating procedure)	1 point
4. Presence of at least 3 diagnosis	1 point	4. Use of laparoscopic technique	-1 point
SENIC score = Σ item 1,2,3,4		NNIS score = Σ item 1,2,3,4	

Table 3. Risk indexes for post-surgical wound infections.

Class	Classification	Infection rate	
		With presurgical antibiotic prophylaxis	Without presurgical antibiotic prophylaxis
Class I	Clean surgery	5.1%	0.8%
Class II	Clean-contaminated surgery	10.1%	1.3%
Class III	Contaminated surgery	21.9%	10.2%
Class IV	Septic surgery		

Table 4. Risk of post-surgical wound infection depending on the Altemeier classification.

3. Management of antibacterial chemotherapeutic drugs

The choice of antibiotics is conditioned by:

- the characteristics of the isolated or suspected aetiological agent,
- patient characteristics, which may influence the efficiency and toxicity of the treatment (age, physiological status, comorbidities, infection site),
- pharmacodynamic and pharmacokinetic characteristics of the antibiotic (adsorption, tissue distribution, concentration in the infectious focus, metabolisation and elimination of the antibiotic).

In the case of the critical patients, the early administration of an effective antibiotic treatment is essential and determining, the time until the initiation of therapy being a strong predictor of mortality. A retrospective cohort study showed that the delay of effective treatment after the onset of recurrent or persistent hypotension was associated with an increased death risk; the survival rate in patients with treatment administered during the first hour was of 79.9%, with each hour of delay in antibiotic therapy leading to a 7.6% decrease in this rate [27].

Optimization of doses. The antibiotic requirement is calculated depending on the characteristics of the patient (age, weight, renal function), on the pathogenic microorganism, infection site (endocarditis, pneumonia, meningitis, osteomyelitis) and the pharmacokinetic and pharmacodynamic characteristics of the drug [28].

The loading dose is probably the most important and depends on the distribution volume of the drug and on the intended plasmatic concentration, regardless of the renal function. Antibiotics are classified according to multiple criteria, one being the criterion, which influences the dosage: the doses of hydrophilic antibiotics (beta-lactam) must be increased during the first stages of sepsis, together with the increase in the extravascular space. The doses of lipophilic antibiotics are influenced by other factors, such as obesity [7, 28].

Before establishing the rational antibiotics administration regimen, the antimicrobial activity in time must be understood, i.e., the pharmacodynamics of the drug in question (the relationship between its serum concentration and its therapeutic effect). From a pharmacodynamic perspective, antimicrobial agents may be divided into:

- The bactericidal effect of beta-lactam antibiotics is independent of their concentration, as long as this exceeds the MIC and they do not possess a significant post-antibiotic effect (PAE) (The inhibition of bacterial growth continued for a variable period after the concentration of antibiotic at the infection site has dropped under the MIC.) The strategy to obtain optimal results is to increase the exposure time of microbes to plasmatic concentrations of antibiotic exceeding the MIC, which is accomplished by frequent doses, by the administration at short time intervals or by continuous infusion.

- The bactericidal effect of vancomycin, carbapenems, macrolides, clindamycin, azoles, linezolid is independent of their concentration, if this is higher than the MIC, but it is time dependent. The PAE is intermediate (The serum antibiotic levels may drop under the MIC for a short while.) The antibiotics in this group produce optimal results when administered in lower but with more frequent doses.

- The bactericidal effect of aminoglycosides, fluoroquinolones and metronidazole is dose dependent and has a significant post-antibiotic effect (Bacterial growth is prevented even if tissue levels decrease under the MIC for longer periods of time.) This is why higher doses, but at larger intervals, may be administered, with 2–4 h between the doses after being admitted, during which time the plasmatic concentration of these antibiotics may be undetectable, which reduces their nephrotoxicity.

The time-dependent bactericidal effect is achieved by optimising the duration of bacterial exposure to antibiotics, while the dose-dependent bactericidal effect is maximal when the antibiotic concentration is maximal [7].

Polymyxins are concentration-dependent antibiotics; they are active on carbapenemase-producing bacteria, and they are increasingly kept as last therapeutic option in infections with resistant pathogens, such as *Pseudomonas aeruginosa*, *Acinetobacter baumannii* and *Klebsiella pneumoniae*. We must underline the fact that if sub-optimal doses of colistin are administered, the pathogen gains resistance.

First-line antibiotic treatment in severe acute infections.

Severe acute infections are classified as community-acquired, healthcare-associated and hospital-acquired infections. For the practical assessment of a case, Yehuda Carmeli proposed a score, which allows the stratification of risk factors for the infections with resistant or MDRO, depending on the previous contact of the patient with the health care sector, on the existence in his/her medical history of antibiotic treatments, as well as on associated factors (immune suppression, co-morbidities):

Risk assessment for infections with resistant or MDR pathogens:

a. Contact with the health care sector:

 1. No contact—1
 2. Contact without invasive procedures—2
 3. Repeated contacts with invasive procedures—3

b. Previous antibiotic treatment:

 1. No antibiotics—1
 2. With antibiotics—2

c. Characteristics of the patient:

 1. Young, without co-morbidities—1
 2. Elderly, with co-morbidities—2
 3. Immunocompromised patient (AIDS, neoplastic diseases)—3

According to this score, the value 1 corresponds to community-acquired infections, the value 2 corresponds to HCAI and the value 3 to hospital-acquired infections. The Carmeli score may only be 1, 2 or 3, and it is given by the highest value obtained from the answers to the three categories of questions [29]. This classification allows a correlation between the type of infection, the most probable aetiology and the estimation of the antibiotic susceptibility of the microorganism in question.

The empirical or first-line treatment is especially important for the evolution of the infection; the delayed initiation of an effective antimicrobial treatment leads to increased morbidity and mortality, aggravated and generalised infections, as well as increased health care costs. If the initial treatment has not been effective, adding a new antibiotic or replacing the initial one with a broader spectrum antibiotic (escalation) will not increase the chance of favourable evolution. The adjustment of antibiotic treatment after the microbiological results become available might be tardy and ineffective, if the initial treatment has been inadequate, especially in the case of hospital-acquired infections (multivariate analysis have demonstrated that inadequate empirical treatment increased the risk of mortality). The association of antibiotics of different classes is useful in the initial treatment of infections with MDRO.

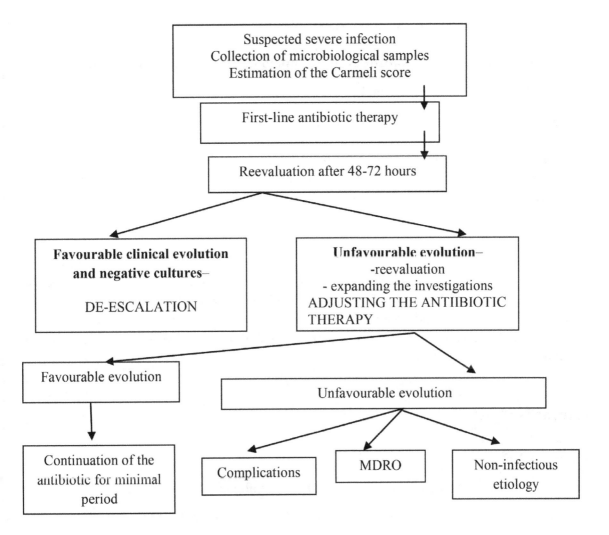

Figure 2. Algorithm for initiation of antibiotic therapy.

In patients with severe infections, the recommendation is to administer the antibiotic treatment during the first hour after the diagnosis, but not before collection of blood and other biological samples required for the identification of the aetiological agent and testing for its sensitivity to chemotherapeutics. Patients with meningitis will receive antibiotic treatment during the first 30 min after hospital admission, immediately after collection of blood and CSF [1, 10].

The empirical or first-line antibiotic treatment is initiated according to the most probable microbiological spectrum and consists of the administration of a broad-spectrum antibiotic (covering Gram-positive cocci, including MRSA and enterococci, as well as Gram-negative bacilli, including *Acinetobacter* spp., *Pseudomonas aeruginosa* and *Enterobacter* spp.) for a short period of time, i.e., for 2–3 days. Depending on the clinical evolution of the patient and on the results of microbiological tests, the initial treatment scheme may be modified by decreasing the number of antibiotics or reducing the spectrum (*de-escalation*). Narrowing the therapeutic regimen does not only refer to the shift from a broad-spectrum to a narrow-spectrum antibiotic, but also to adjusting (reducing) the doses and treatment duration [30].

The Principles of de-escalation are as follows:

- administration of an ultra-broad-spectrum antibiotic for a short period of time,
- identification of the aetiology within this covered period,
- replacement of the initial antibiotic with a narrow-spectrum antibiotic.

If, after 48–72 h of treatment with a broad-spectrum antibiotic, the status of the patient does not improve, the available microbiological data are attentively reanalysed and the possibility of MDRO infection, a non-bacterial or even a non-infectious aetiology, are considered. The evaluation must also include the possibility of a complication, such as the formation of an abscess, empyema, etc. [31].

Decreasing the risk of adverse reactions, the decreased selection pressure of resistant strains, as well as the reduction of costs represent the benefits of de-escalation and treatment cessation after a shorter time. Examples of benefits in the administration of antibiotics in short cures and/or reduction of the antibiotics spectrum include the decrease in the incidence of cases of diarrhoea with *Clostridium difficile* and of infections with resistant bacteria and *Candida* spp. (**Figure 2**).

Author details

Muntean Delia and Licker Monica*

*Address all correspondence to: deliacristimuntean@yahoo.com

"Victor Babes" University of Medicine and Pharmacy, Timisoara, Romania

References

[1] Niederman MS, Craven DE, Bonten MJ, et al. Guidelines for the management of adults with hospital-acquired, ventilator-associated, and healthcare-associated pneumonia. American Journal of Respiratory and Critical Care Medicine. 2005;**171**:388-416

[2] Marin H, Kollef MLE, Baughman RP. Health care-associated pneumonia (HCAP): A critical appraisal to improve identification, management, and outcomes-proceedings of the HCAP summit. Clinical Infectious Diseases. 2008;**46**(Supl 4):S296-S334

[3] Rello J, Kollef M, Diaz E, Rodriguez A. Infectious Diseases in Critical Care. Berlin Heidelberg: Springer-Verlag; 2007. pp. 203-205

[4] https://publications.europa.eu/ro/publication-detail/-/publication/10ed460f-0711-11e2-8e28-01aa75ed71a1/language-ro

[5] ***CDC Bacterial Pneumonia, MMWR. 1997;**46**:RR1-RR85

[6] Strausbaugh LJ. Nosocomial respiratory infections. In: Mandell GL, Bennett JE, Mandell Douglas DR, Bennett's, editors. Principles and Practice of Infectious Diseases. 6th ed. Vol. 2005. Elsevier Churchill Livingstone. pp. 3362-3369

[7] Rello J. Importance of appropriate initial antibiotic therapy and deescaladation in the treatment of nosocomial pneumonia. European Respiratory Review. 2007;**16**(103):33-39

[8] Burke AC: Bacterial sepsis. 2011. Available from: http://misc.medscape.com/pi/android/medscapeapp/html/A234587-business.html

[9] Mackenzie I, Lever A. Management of sepsis. BMJ. 2007;**335**(7626):929-932

[10] Micek ST, Welch EC, et al. Empiric combination antibiotic therapy is associated with improved outcome against sepsis due to gram-negative bacteria: A retrospective analysis. Antimicrobial Agents and Chemotherapy. 2010;**54**(5):1742-1748

[11] Lim LM, Neang Ly BS, Anderson D, et al. Resurgence of Colistin: A review of resistance, toxicity, pharmacodynamics and dosing. Pharmacotherapy. 2010;**30**(12):1279-1291

[12] Arnold RS, Thom KA, Sharma S, et al. Emergence of *Klebsiella pneumoniae* carbapenemase-producing bacteria. Southern Medical Journal. 2011;**104**(1):40-45

[13] Lee J, Patel G, Huprikar S, et al. Decreased susceptibility to polymyxin B during treatment of carbapenem-resistant *Klebsiella pneumonia* infection. Journal of Clinical Microbiology. 2009;**47**:1611-1612

[14] Wagenlehne FM, Pilatz A, Naber KG, Weidner W. Therapeutic challenges of urosepsis. European Journal of Clinical Investigation. 2008;**38**(S2):45-49

[15] Barsiç B, Beus E, Marton E, et al. Nosocomial infections in critically ill infectious diseases patients: Results of a 7-year focal surveillance. Infection. 1999;**27**(1):20-26

[16] Beekmann SE, Henderson DK. Infections caused by percutaneous intravascular devices. In: Mandell GL, Bennett JE, Mandell Douglas DR, Bennett's, editors. Principles and Practice of Infectious Diseases. 6th ed. Elsevier Churchill Livingstone; 2005. pp. 3347-3360

[17] ***CDC Guideline for Prevention of Cateter-Related Nosocomial Infections. Vol. 51. MMWR; 2002. p. RR10

[18] Fernandez-Hidalgo N. Antibiotic-lock therapy for long-term intravascular catheter-related bacteraemia: Results of an open, non-comparative study. The Journal of Antimicrobial Chemotherapy. 2006;**57**(6):1172-1180

[19] Gupta K, Hooton TM, Naber KG, et al. International clinical practice guidelines for the treatment of acute uncomplicated cystitis and pyelonephritis in women: A 2010 update by the Infectious Diseases Society of America and the European Society for Microbiology and Infectious Diseases. Clinical Infectious Diseases. 2011;**52**(5):e103-e120

[20] http://uroweb.org/wp-content/uploads/Guidelines_WebVersion_Complete-1.pdf

[21] Hopkins J. Antibiotic Guidelines 2015-2016. Treatment Recommendations for Adult Inpatients. Available from: insidehopkinsmedicine.org/amp

[22] Sartelli M. A focus on intra-abdominal infections. World Journal of Emergency Surgery. 2010;**5**:9

[23] Brouwer MC, Tunkel AR, van de Beek D. Epidemiology, diagnosis, and antimicrobial treatment of acute bacterial meningitis. Clinical Microbiology Reviews. 2010;**23**(3):467-492

[24] Nau R, Sörgel F, Eiffert H. Penetration of drugs through the blood-cerebrospinal fluid/blood-brain barrier for treatment of central nervous system infections. Clinical Microbiology Reviews. 2010;**23**(4):858-883

[25] Rajan S. Skin and soft-tissue infections: Classifying and treating a spectrum. Cleveland Clin J Med. 2012;**79**(1):57-66

[26] Talbot TR, Kaiser AB. Postoperative infections and antimicrobial prophylaxis. In: Mandell GL, Bennett JE, Mandell Douglas DR, Bennett's, editors. Principles and Practice of Infectious Diseases. 6th ed. Elsevier Churchill Livingstone; 2005. pp. 3533-3344

[27] Kumar A, Roberts D, Wood KE, et al. Duration of hypotension before initiation of effective antimicrobial therapy is the critical determinant of survival in human septic shock. Critical Care Medicine. 2006;**34**:1589-1596

[28] Morrell MR, Micek ST, Kollef MH. The management of severe sepsis and septic shock. Infectious Disease Clinics of North America. 2009;**23**(3):485-501

[29] Carmeli Y. The Role of Carbapenems: The Predictive Factors for Multi-Drug–Resistant Gram-Negatives. 2006. Available from: www.invanz.co.il/

[30] Kollef MH, Ward S, Sherman G, et al. Inadequate treatment of nosocomial infections is associated with certain empiric antibiotic choices. Critical Care Medicine. 2000;**28**:3456-3364

[31] Deresinski S. Principles of antibiotic therapy in severe infections: Optimizing the therapeutic approach by use of laboratory and clinical data. Clinical Infectious Diseases. 2007;**45**(supl 3):S177-S183

Acute Kidney Injury in the Intensive Care Unit

Jose J. Zaragoza and Faustino J. Renteria

Abstract

Acute kidney injury (AKI) is defined as an abrupt decrease in glomerular filtration rate (GFR). Incidence varies from 20% to as high as 70% in critically ill patients. Classically, AKI has been divided into three broad pathophysiologic categories: prerenal AKI, intrinsic AKI, and postrenal (obstructive) AKI. The clinical manifestations of AKI vary among a wide range of symptoms and metabolic abnormalities. A sudden decrease in GFR will result in rising concentrations of solutes in the blood, which are normally excreted by the kidneys. Recently, new urinary and serum biomarkers have gained a place in the diagnosis, classification, and prognosis prediction of AKI. The best treatment for AKI is prevention. Patients with prerenal azotemia should have intravascular volume deficits corrected and cardiac function optimized. Obstructive (postrenal) kidney disease is treated by mechanical relief of the block. The primary management of acute interstitial nephritis is discontinuation of the inciting agent. Renal replacement therapy (RRT) has emerged as a supportive mechanism rather than just as a lifesaving measure. Continuous techniques are preferable in treating critically ill patients, although every modality has its benefits, indications, and contraindications.

Keywords: acute kidney injury, acute renal failure, intensive care unit, glomerular filtration rate, renal replacement therapy

1. Introduction

Acute kidney injury (AKI) is now recognized as a major health problem that affects millions of patients worldwide and leads to decreased survival and increased risk of progression to chronic kidney disease (CKD). It is often diagnosed along with other acute illnesses and is common in critically ill patients. AKI has also an important role since it is strongly associated with augmented costs of care, worse outcomes, and diminished quality of life after discharge. The impact and prognosis of AKI vary considerably depending on the severity, clinical setting, comorbid factors, and geographical location [1].

AKI in the ICU is common, and it is increasing in incidence. Reported mortality in ICU patients with AKI varies between studies depending on AKI definition and the patient population studied. In most studies, mortality increases proportionately with increasing severity of AKI. In patients with severe AKI requiring renal replacement therapy (RRT), mortality is approximately 50–70%. Although AKI requiring RRT in the ICU is a well-recognized independent risk factor for in-hospital mortality, even small changes in serum creatinine (SCr) are associated with increased mortality.

The definition of AKI has many perceptions, the simplest way to describe it is as a sudden decrease in glomerular filtration rate (GFR) resulting in the retention of metabolic waste products and the dysregulation of fluid, electrolyte and acid-base homeostasis. AKI is a heterogeneous syndrome that includes hemodynamic disarrangements that disturb normal renal perfusion and decrease GFR without overt parenchymal injury; partial or complete obstruction to urine flow; and acute parenchymal injury resulting in glomerular, interstitial, tubular, or vascular dysfunction. The most common causes of AKI in critically ill patients include hemodynamically mediated prerenal dysfunction and acute tubular necrosis (ATN) due to ischemia-reperfusion injury, nephrotoxic exposure, or sepsis [2].

The cardinal manifestation of AKI is the retention of metabolic waste products, most commonly represented by creatinine and urea, and/or fluid accumulation. More than 35 clinical definitions of AKI currently exist in the literature. The Acute Dialysis Quality Initiative convened in 2002 and proposed the RIFLE classification (risk, injury, failure, loss, end-stage kidney disease) specifically for AKI in critically ill patients. Using SCr and urine output, the RIFLE criteria define three grades of severity and two outcome classes. Later, the Acute Kidney Injury Network (AKIN) proposed another clinical and practical definition. Even small changes in serum creatinine concentrations are associated with a substantial increase in the risk of death. For this reason, in 2012, the Kidney Disease Improving Global Outcomes (KDIGO) classification defined AKI as a raise of serum creatinine of at least 0.3 mg/dl or as a urine output of less than 0.3 ml/kg/h for at least 6 h (**Table 1**) [3].

2. Epidemiology

The epidemiology of AKI varies depending on the type and characteristics of the population described. Using the current 0.3-mg/dl change in serum creatinine threshold, published data ranges the incidence of AKI in hospitalized patients from 3 to 50% and from 10 to 70% in the intensive care unit (ICU). A 2013 meta-analysis of AKI incidence per the kidney improving global outcomes staging system with a total number of patients included of 3,585,911, reported incidence in 23% overall hospitalized patients [4].

Stage	RIFLE	AKIN	KDIGO	Urine output
RIFLE–Risk AKIN/ KDIGO Stage 1	Increase in serum creatinine × 1.5 (within 7 days)	Increase in serum creatinine of 0.3 mg/dl or > × 1.5 (within 48 h)	Increase in serum creatinine of 0.3 mg/dl (within 48 h) or × 1.5 (within 7 days)	Urine output of < 0.5 mg/kg/h for > 6 h
RIFLE–Injury AKIN/ KDIGO Stage 2	Increase in serum creatinine × 2	Increase in serum creatinine × 2	Increase in serum creatinine × 2	Urine output of < 0.5 mg/kg/h for > 12 h
RIFLE–Failure AKIN/ KDIGO Stage 3	Increase in serum creatinine × 3 or above 4.0 mg/dl	Increase in serum creatinine × 3 or above 4.0 mg/dl	Increase in serum creatinine × 3 or above 4.0 mg/dl	Urine output of < 0.3 mg/kg/h for > 24 h or anuria for > 12 h
RIFLE–Loss	Need for RRT for >4 weeks			
RIFLE–End stage	Need for RRT for >3 months			

Table 1. AKI definition by clinical parameters per RIFLE, AKIN, and KDIGO.

Among critically ill patients, numerous cohort studies have been issued to define the incidence of AKI in ICU. Final reports suggest that it goes as high as 70% in some populations. Patients with ICU-associated AKI are younger, more likely to be male and prone to have AKI associated with multisystem organ failure as opposed to isolated AKI. The most important recognized risk factor for AKI in the ICU environment is sepsis. Other important risk factors include previous diagnosis of Diabetes, Hypertension or CKD, concomitant use of vasopressors and use of mechanical ventilation. Renal replacement therapy (RRT) rates and mortality associated to AKI are significantly higher among ICU population opposed to hospitalized patients [5].

Two distinct patterns of ICU-associated AKI have been described: community-acquired AKI, present at ICU admission, and hospital-acquired AKI. Patients with hospital-acquired AKI have more severe outcomes, showing higher in-hospital mortality rates, longer lengths of stay both in the ICU and hospital, and higher needs of RRT [6, 7].

3. Pathophysiology

AKI can be divided into three broad etiologic categories: prerenal AKI, intrinsic AKI, and postrenal (**Figure 1**). Prerenal refers to states of hypoperfusion of the kidneys without a parenchymal damage, this kind of AKI occurs often in ICU patients. Postrenal or obstructive AKI is characterized by acute block of the urinary tract. Regarding intrinsic dysfunction, acute damage to the renal parenchyma exists, as in acute tubular necrosis, acute interstitial nephritis and/or acute glomerular nephritis. The terms "prerenal," "intrinsic," and "postrenal" are used to group common pathophysiologic features and not diagnosis. It was a long-held view that "prerenal AKI" or "transient" AKI were synonymous with "hypovolemic AKI" and "fluid responsiveness," this is no longer the case and must not be used in this manner. Approach to the diagnosis and treatment is described below [8, 9].

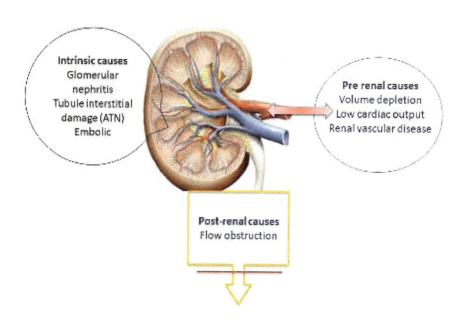

Figure 1. Traditional etiologic categories for AKI.

3.1. Prerenal AKI

Prerenal AKI is the most common pathophysiologic cause of AKI, contributing to the development 30–60% of all cases of AKI in ICU. Prerenal AKI develops when the capacity of the normal physiologic responses to hypovolemia is exceeded. This response initiates with a decrease in mean arterial pressure, triggering baroreceptors that lead the activation of the sympathetic nervous system, activation of the renin-angiotensin-aldosterone system (RAAS), and secretion of the antidiuretic hormone vasopressin. The activation of the renal sympathetic nerves constricts the afferent (preglomerular) arterioles and stimulates release of renin from the juxtaglomerular apparatus. Renin secretion is also directly stimulated in response to hypovolemia by changes in intrarenal hemodynamic. Secretion of renin activates a cascade with the final production of angiotensin II. Angiotensin II stimulates both afferent and efferent (postglomerular) arteriolar vasoconstriction; however, the effect on the afferent vessel is opposed by vasodilatory prostaglandins, kallikrein, kinins, and nitric oxide. The net effect is vasoconstriction of both afferent and efferent arterioles and decrease of GFR to maintain circulating volume at near normal levels by the production of concentrated urine with low sodium content (i.e., fractional excretion of sodium) [10–12].

In classic forms of prerenal AKI, reduced renal perfusion pressure (or increased renal venous pressure) and afferent arteriolar constriction combined lower the glomerular capillary hydrostatic pressure below the autoregulation capacity and consequently the net ultrafiltration pressure, hence diminishing GFR. Prerenal AKI may be caused by extracellular fluid volume loss or shifts, reduced cardiac output, systemic vasodilation, intrarenal vasoconstriction, or increased renal venous pressure.

3.2. Renal AKI

Intrinsic AKI is commonly divided into tubular, interstitial, glomerular, and vascular processes depending on the nephron region that is the most affected. The most common intrinsic cause of AKI is ATN, accounting for 85–90% of intrinsic ICU-associated AKI. The causes of ATN can be broken down into three major categories: ischemia-reperfusion injury, nephrotoxic, and septic. Sepsis-associated ATN has unique features and may develop in the absence of overt renal ischemia [13].

3.2.1. Sepsis-associated ATN

Sepsis has long been recognized as a foremost precipitant of AKI and deserves a distinction. Sepsis-associated AKI (SA-AKI) portends a high burden of morbidity and mortality in both children and adults with critical illness. Observational data suggest that injury during SA-AKI occurs early of the critical illness and after ICU admission. In a large recent cohort, 68% of 5443 patients with septic shock had evidence of AKI within 6 h after presentation. The development of AKI later during an episode of sepsis has been associated with worse clinical outcome and increased mortality rates (76.5 vs. 61.5% in early AKI) [14].

Sepsis-mediated hypo perfusion leading to tubular necrosis has been traditionally cited as the main pathophysiology for SA-AKI; however, mounting evidence has challenged this paradigm. Numerous drivers for injury now are recognized as playing a role in SA-AKI, including ischemia-reperfusion injury, nephron inflammation, hypoxic and/or oxidant stress, cytokine and chemokine-driven direct tubular injury, and tubular and mesenchymal apoptosis. For instance, renal vein thermodilution measurement of RBF in eight septic critically ill patients did not show hypoperfusion to the glomerulus consistently. Tubular cellular injury contributes to the propagation of AKI during sepsis. Several causal mechanisms appear to be involved, but tubular necrosis, traditionally cited as the major cellular switch for injury, is not supported by the available experimental evidence. Renal tubular apoptosis in response to the stress of systemic sepsis now is cited as a potential contributing mechanism of injury in SA-AKI [14–16].

Similarly, cellular hypoxia is a molecular driver of injury during SA-AKI. Tissue hypoxia in the kidney during sepsis may be defined by inflammation, changes in intrarenal nitric oxide, nitrosative stress or oxygen radical homeostasis, and dysregulation. Downregulation of mediators of oxidative phosphorylation occurs during sepsis and protection of mitochondrial respiration may mitigate renal injury during sepsis [14, 17, 18].

3.3. Postrenal AKI

AKI resulting from obstruction usually causes fewer than 5% of ICU-associated AKI. Obstruction above the level of the bladder is referred to as upper tract obstruction. The development of AKI from upper tract obstruction requires the presence of bilateral obstruction or unilateral obstruction in the setting of a single functioning kidney or dysfunction of the contralateral kidney.

Patients with obstructive disease may present with anuria if obstruction is complete, with normal or increased urine volume in a partial obstruction, or with fluctuating urine output with periods of anuria alternating with rapid passage of urine as the pressure in the collecting system rises and overcomes the block. In the acute phase of obstruction, intratubular pressure rises over venous renal pressure replacing the latter in the net filtration pressure equation. When intratubular pressure reaches close to mean arterial pressure, net filtration pressure falls below the autoregulation range, sometimes almost to zero [19].

4. Clinical findings

The clinical manifestations of AKI vary from a wide range of signs and symptoms. The syndrome encompasses from laboratory abnormalities without symptoms to organ failure exhibiting fluid overload and severe electrolyte and/or acid-base disturbances [20].

A sudden decrease in GFR results in rising concentrations of waste products, commonly represented by urea end creatinine in the blood. The relationship between the GFR and the concentration of urea and creatinine in blood stream is nonlinear and may be affected by a variety of other factors. The level of blood urea nitrogen (BUN) generally correlates with the symptoms, with uremic manifestations usually absent until the BUN is above 100 mg/dl. Creatinine is derived from the nonenzymatic hydrolysis of creatine, which is usually released at a constant rate from skeletal muscle and is excreted primarily by filtration at the glomerulus. There is essentially no tubular reabsorption of creatinine. That is why, in the absence of glomerular filtration, serum creatinine typically increases by 1–2 mg/dl/day. The role of creatinine as a marker of renal function is limited by the fact that the serum concentration may take 24–36 h to rise after a renal insult. Additionally, ICU patients commonly accumulate fluid due to intravenous administration and concomitant AKI. Fluid overload decreases creatinine concentration since it dilutes the total amount of creatinine in the extracellular fluid. A true change in GFR may not be adequately reflected by serum creatinine in patients with sepsis, liver disease, fluid overload, and/or muscle wasting [20].

Urine output of less than 400–500 ml/day or a sustained urine output of less than 20 ml/h in a high-risk patient in the absence of volume depletion almost always indicates the presence of AKI. By KDIGO definition, a urine output of less than 0.5 ml/kg/h for 6 h indicates the occurrence of AKI [3].

4.1. Biomarkers

Cystatin C is a cysteine protease inhibitor that is released into the bloodstream at a constant rate from all nucleated cells. It is filtered at the glomerulus and reabsorbed and catabolized by renal proximal tubular epithelial cells such that virtually no cystatin C appears in the urine. The interindividual variability in cystatin C production appears to be less than that for creatinine. Cystatin C may be a more reliable marker of GFR [21].

Several relatively new biomarkers of tubular injury have been proposed as novel diagnostic tests for the early diagnosis of AKI. These markers include kidney injury molecule-1 (KIM-1), neutrophil gelatinase-associated lipocalin (NGAL), interleukin 18 (IL-18), liver fatty acid binding protein (L-FABP), and α- and π-glutathione-S-transferase (GST), among others. They have been tested particularly amid cardiac surgery patients, with good predicting values. Even though these markers seem promising, these are not suitable for indiscriminate use in every ICU patient, and their exact specific role at the bedside remains uncertain [22, 23].

A novel test method measures two small tubular cell–derived molecules, Insulin-like Growth Factor Binding Protein 7 (IGFBP7) and Tissue Inhibitor of Metalloproteinase 2 (TIMP-2). IGFBP7 and TIMP-2 are markers of cell cycle arrest and possibly apoptosis, inflammation, and tubular cell repair. The above-stated conditions appear to be the most relevant in the development of tubular cell injury, when the loss of cell polarity, brush border derangement, and cell sloughing might occur. Such injury may deflect the organism from normal repair toward maladaptive and lead to CKD, which further predisposes the individual to recurrent AKI [24].

According to recently published data, this test possesses the highest sensitivity for detecting AKI at an early stage. The Astute140™ meter is a device based on a fluorescence labeling technique, which detects fluorescent signals from the immunoassay and calculates concentrations of IGFBP7 and TIMP-2 from the inserted cartridge. The device converts the measured signals into a single number, defining the relative risk of the patient developing AKI. The result, known as the AKIRisk score, is obtained within 20 min [25].

5. Approach

The first step in evaluating a patient with AKI in the ICU is to determine whether kidney hypo perfusion plays a role in the current state. Physical examination should focus on assessing for evidence of volume depletion, such as dry mucous membranes, decreased skin turgor, and absence of sweat in the axilla and inguinal regions. If necessary, a more complete assessment should be done before or at the ICU. Advance hemodynamic monitoring is reasonable in high-risk patients, particularly using dynamic measurements of cardiac function, or even a complete ultrasound and echocardiographic evaluation at the bedside [26].

Placement of a bladder catheter should be performed to exclude urethra obstruction as a cause of AKI, but primarily, to initiate real-time urinary flow monitoring. Urinary output express information of whether our actions and treatment result in the patients' improvement. Urinary sediment should be examined under the microscope to discard other causes of AKI, especially intrinsic causes. In the presence of proteinuria, a urinary sediment containing abundant cells or casts suggests an intrinsic cause of AKI rather than hypoperfusion as the primary mechanism. Precisely, the presence of renal tubular epithelial cells, epithelial cell casts, or pigmented (muddy brown) granular casts suggests the diagnosis of ATN and is associated with the increased risk for bad outcomes. A normal urine sediment suggests the presence of either a prerenal or postrenal pathophysiology of AKI, although obstructive uropathy may be associated with haematuria, pyuria, or crystalluria. The electrolyte composition of the urine may be helpful in differentiating between prerenal and ATN (i.e., fractional excretion of sodium), but not to guide the treatment [27, 28].

Imaging of the kidneys and bladder is required for the diagnosis of obstructive kidney disease and might provide information about the prehospital kidney function. Enlarged kidneys in a diabetic patient suggest that a previous damage was present, and GFR was diminished at baseline. This is especially helpful in a community-acquired AKI patient in whose previous renal function is unknown.

5.1. Clinical vs. subclinical AKI

The pitfalls of currently recommended diagnosis of AKI (i.e. creatinine and urinary flow) and the discovery of the above-mentioned new biomarkers have created new insights in AKI approach. The alteration of tubular and cellular arrest biomarkers, without creatinine elevation or a diminish of urinary flow, has led to the theory that at least some of the nephrons in the kidneys have suffered damage despite lack of azotemia (i.e. subclinical AKI). New classification for AKI has been proposed based on this. This new classification encompasses both clinical (i.e., with elevation in creatinine) and subclinical (i.e., alteration in biomarkers without creatinine elevation) AKI (**Figure 2**) [3, 23].

6. Treatment

The best treatment for AKI is acknowledging the existing risk factors and prevention. Diminish the time of hypo perfusion in every patient with AKI by a rapid recognition of cardiac output deficits, keeping an adequate intravascular effective volume and avoid nephrotoxic are keystones of prevention.

There is no specific management that accommodates the clear majority of patients with established AKI. Patients with prerenal AKI, as mentioned, should have intravascular volume deficits corrected and cardiac function optimized. Obstructive (postrenal) kidney disease is treated by mechanical relief of the obstruction. The primary management of acute interstitial

Type of AKI	Creatinine BUN	Urine Output	Biomarkers
Clinical AKI	↑	↓	↓
Subclinical AKI	↓	↑	↑

Figure 2. Clinical vs. subclinical AKI.

nephritis is discontinuation of the inciting agent; in patients with persistent AKI, there may be a role for treatment with glucocorticoids.

Once volume status and cardiac output have been optimized, if the patient remains oliguric, the use of a unique trial of diuretics to establish urine output can be considered. Although nonoliguric forms of ATN are associated with significantly lower risk of morbidity and mortality than oliguric forms, the primary rationale for a trial of diuretic therapy is to facilitate volume management not to improve AKI. None of the most common diuretics used in ICU worldwide increase the GFR. Positive fluid balance after development of AKI is associated with increased mortality rate, and avoiding fluid accumulation has a protective effect over mortality. The use of renal vasodilators, including dopamine, fenoldopam, and atrial natriuretic peptide, has not been shown to be beneficial in AKI, and its use should be discouraged [3].

AKI is associated with the development of sometimes serious electrolyte and acid-base disturbances, including hyperkalemia, hyponatremia, hyperphosphatemia, hypo- and (less commonly) hypercalcemia, hypermagnesemia, hyperuricemia, and metabolic acidosis. In addition, AKI is associated with anemia, bleeding diatheses, increased risk of infections, and dysfunction of other organ systems, including cardiovascular dysfunction, respiratory failure, gastrointestinal complications, and neurologic disturbances. These complications should be in mind of the treating physician in the ICU at every time [29, 30].

6.1. Renal replacement therapy

In patients with severe AKI, RRT is the cornerstone of supportive management. One objective of RRT includes allowing the removal of fluid and solutes that accumulate during renal failure. The available modalities of RRT comprise intermittent hemodialysis (IHD), the various forms of continuous renal replacement therapy (CRRT), and the hybrid modalities of prolonged intermittent RRT (PIRRT; also, extended duration dialysis [EDD] or sustained low-efficiency dialysis [SLED]) [31, 32].

Solute removal during RRT may occur by diffusion down a concentration gradient from the blood across a semipermeable membrane into dialysate or by convective transport of solute across the membrane during filtration. Fluid removal occurs by filtration, driven by either a hydrostatic or osmotic pressure gradient across the semipermeable membrane. In conventional IHD, the patient's blood passes through a semipermeable hemodialyzer counter current to the flow of dialysate on the other side of the membrane. The dialysis solution has a composition that approximates the normal electrolyte conformation of extracellular fluids and creates equilibrium to the blood, normalizing solutes. CRRT utilizes either diffusive hemodialysis, convective hemofiltration, or a combination of both. In addition to the duration of therapy, the major difference between intermittent and continuous hemodialysis is the dialysate flow rate. In intermittent hemodialysis, dialysate flow rates (typically 500–800 ml/min) are equal to or greater than blood flow rates, allowing rapid solute clearance. In continuous hemodialysis, the dialysate flow rate (typically 15–30 ml/min) is slow compared to that of the blood, permitting virtual equilibration of low-molecular-weight solutes such as urea between the blood and dialysate. Thus, solute clearance for low-molecular-weight solutes approximates the dialysate flow rate. Nonetheless, the total daily or weekly clearance is greater with continuous treatment, due to the extended time of therapy.

In continuous hemofiltration, a high filtration rate is generated, and physiologic replacement fluid is administered at an equal rate. Negative fluid balance (ultrafiltration) is accomplished by administering less milliliter per hour (usually 50–400 ml/h). Solute removal occurs exclusively by convection, and clearance is approximately equal to the ultrafiltration rate. The convective transport is limited primarily by the pore size of the membrane, so hemofiltration provides more efficient clearance of higher molecular weight (>500–15,000 KDa) solutes. Although it has been proposed that removal of higher molecular weight solutes with hemofiltration as compared to hemodialysis would be of clinical benefit, this has not been borne out in clinical trials. Because of their prolonged duration, the net ultrafiltration rate required to attain the same daily fluid removal is lower with CRRT than with IHD. Thus, CRRT is generally considered to cause less hemodynamic instability than conventional IHD [33].

Finally, PIRRT is a modification of conventional IHD, utilizing lower blood and dialysate flow rates while prolonging the treatment duration to 8–16 h.

There has been considerable debate regarding which modality is most appropriate for use in critically ill patients with AKI. Current data suggest that no individual modality of RRT provides either better patient survival or recovery of kidney function. These modalities should be complementary and must not be considered as mutually exclusive. According to the KDIGO guidelines, CRRT must be considered the first-line treatment in hemodynamically unstable patients and those with neurological illness whom require RRT and might be prone to develop cerebral edema [3].

Conventional indications for initiation of RRT include volume overload unresponsive to diuretic therapy, electrolyte and acid-base disturbances refractory to medical management, severe hyperkalemia, metabolic acidosis, overt uremia, characterized pericarditis, or encephalopathy. Most of the AKI patients in the ICU do not spent enough time in the hospital to express most of these indications. Initiating RRT in a patient with some of the conventional indications is unquestionable, although the use in other cases when the alterations do not endanger life immediately is uncertain. Studies have shown conflictive results when comparing the so-called early and late initiation strategies, with no clear benefit from one over the other. Even, there is no definition of either of them. Benefits of connecting a specific patient should be opposed to the risks of the same action, and each case should be individualized. Keep in mind, the potential harms of connecting too early include unnecessary exposure to the risks related to the catheter insertion, diminishing intravascular effective volume (especially in IHD), and resources utilization that increase costs. The unwanted adverse effect of taking too long in initiating might be death [34].

7. Outcomes

The mortality rate increases with AKI, independently associated to the underlying disease and baseline characteristics. Much higher mortality rates are associated with intrinsic forms of AKI over

[18] Heyman SN, Evans RG, Rosen S, Rosenberger C. Cellular adaptive changes in AKI: Mitigating renal hypoxic injury. Nephrology Dialysis Transplantation 2012;**27**:1721-1728. DOI: 10.1093/ndt/gfs100

[19] Liaño F, Junco E, Pascual J, Madero R, Verde E. The spectrum of acute renal failure in the intensive care unit compared with that seen in other settings. The Madrid Acute Renal Failure Study Group. Kidney International. 1998;**66**:S16-S24

[20] Thomas ME, Blaine C, Dawnay A, Devonald MAJ, Ftouh S, Laing C, et al. The definition of acute kidney injury and its use in practice. Kidney International. 2015;**87**:62-73. DOI: 10.1038/ki.2014.328

[21] Inker LA, Schmid CH, Tighiouart H, Eckfeldt JH, Feldman HI, Greene T, et al. Estimating glomerular filtration rate from serum creatinine and cystatin C. The New England Journal of Medicine 2012;**367**:20-29. DOI: 10.1056/NEJMoa1114248

[22] Han WK, Bailly V, Abichandani R, Thadhani R, Bonventre J V. Kidney Injury Molecule-1 (KIM-1): A novel biomarker for human renal proximal tubule injury. Kidney International. 2002;**62**:237-244. DOI: 10.1046/j.1523-1755.2002.00433.x

[23] Koyner JL, Vaidya VS, Bennett MR, Ma Q, Worcester E, Akhter SA, et al. Urinary biomarkers in the clinical prognosis and early detection of acute kidney injury. Clinical Journal of the American Society of Nephrology 2010;**5**:2154-2165. DOI: 10.2215/CJN.00740110

[24] Aregger F, Uehlinger DE, Witowski J, Brunisholz RA, Hunziker P, Frey FJ, et al. Identification of IGFBP-7 by urinary proteomics as a novel prognostic marker in early acute kidney injury. Kidney International. 2014;**85**:909-919. DOI: 10.1038/ki.2013.363

[25] Pajenda S, Ilhan-Mutlu A, Preusser M, Roka S, Druml W, Wagner L. NephroCheck data compared to serum creatinine in various clinical settings. BMC Nephrology 2015;**16**:206. DOI: 10.1186/s12882-015-0203-5

[26] McGee S, Abernethy WB, Simel DL. The rational clinical examination: Is this patient hypovolemic? Journal of the American Medical Association. 1999;**281**:1022-1029.

[27] Chawla LS, Dommu A, Berger A, Shih S, Patel SS. Urinary sediment cast scoring index for acute kidney injury: A pilot study. Nephron Clinical Practice. 2008;**110**:c145-c150. DOI: 10.1159/000166605

[28] Singer E, Elger A, Elitok S, Kettritz R, Nickolas TL, Barasch J, et al. Urinary neutrophil gelatinase-associated lipocalin distinguishes pre-renal from intrinsic renal failure and predicts outcomes. Kidney International. 2011;**80**:405-414. DOI: 10.1038/ki.2011.41

[29] Zaragoza JJ, Villa G, Garzotto F, Sharma A, Lorenzin A, Ribeiro L, et al. Initiation of renal replacement therapy in the intensive care unit in Vicenza (IRRIV) score. Blood Purification. 2015;**39**:246-257. DOI: 10.1159/000381009

[30] Wald R, Bagshaw SM. The timing of renal replacement therapy initiation in acute kidney injury: Is earlier truly better?. Critical Care Medicine. 2014;**42**:1933-1934. DOI: 10.1097/CCM.0000000000000432

[31] Ronco C, Cruz D, Bellomo R. Continuous renal replacement in critical illness. Contributions to Nephrology. 2007;**156**:309-319. DOI: 10.1159/0000102121

[32] Marshall MR, Golper TA, Shaver MJ, Alam MG, Chatoth DK. Sustained low-efficiency dialysis for critically ill patients requiring renal replacement therapy. Kidney International. 2001;**60**:777-785. DOI: 10.1046/j.1523-1755.2001.060002777.x

[33] Ronco C, Ricci Z, De Backer D, Kellum JA, Taccone FS, Joannidis M, et al. Renal replacement therapy in acute kidney injury: Controversy and consensus. Critical Care. 2015;**19**:146. DOI: 10.1186/s13054-015-0850-8

[34] Joannidis M, Forni LG. Clinical review: Timing of renal replacement therapy. Critical Care 2011;**15**:223. DOI: 10.1186/cc10109

[35] Manns B, Doig CJ, Lee H, Dean S, Tonelli M, Johnson D, et al. Cost of acute renal failure requiring dialysis in the intensive care unit: Clinical and resource implications of renal recovery. Critical Care Medicine 2003;**31**:449-455. DOI: 10.1097/01.CCM.0000045182.90302.B3

[36] Lewers DT, Mathew TH, Maher JF, Schreiner GE. Long-term follow-up of renal function and histology after acute tubular necrosis. Annals of Internal Medicine. 1970;**73**:523. DOI: 10.7326/0003-4819-73-4-523

Measuring and Managing Fluid Overload in Pediatric Intensive Care Unit

Dyah Kanya Wati

Abstract

Fluid management is one of the regular aspects of care in pediatric intensive care unit (PICU) setting, and its importance has been stressed in previous studies. Fluid resuscitation, as part of fluid management, may be needed to maintain intravascular volume, and prior studies showed that early aggressive fluid resuscitation may improve outcome in critical illness, especially in endothelial-dysfunction associated conditions. Unfortunately, this routine management often leads to the development of positive fluid balance and, consequently, fluid overload. Many evidences have stated that excessive fluid administration is closely associated with negative effects for children who were admitted in PICU. Moreover, fluid balance before PICU admission is also important because uncertainty about quantification fluid balance before admission can lead to underestimated fluid overload.

Keywords: positive fluid balance, children, pediatric intensive care, managing

1. Introduction

Fluid management is one of the regular aspects of care in PICU setting, and its importance has been stressed in previous studies [1]. Fluid resuscitation, as part of fluid management, may be needed to maintain intravascular volume [2], and prior studies showed that early aggressive fluid resuscitation may improve outcome in critical illness [1], especially in endothelial-dysfunction associated conditions [3]. Unfortunately, this routine management often leads to the development positive fluid balance and consequently, fluid overload (FO) [1, 3, 4]. Many evidences have stated that excessive fluid administration is closely associated with negative effects for children who were admitted in PICU [3, 4]. FO was known to cause increased risk of morbidity, mortality, additional time of mechanical ventilation, additional hospitalization time, and increased need for renal replacement therapy (RRT) [5, 6].

In patients who already have critically ill also shown that fluid overload shows a negative effect. Flori et al. [2] conducted post-hoc study about the association positive fluid balance with worse clinical outcomes in children with ALI. This study showed the increment of 10 mL/kg/day fluid balance was associated with increasing mortality. Moreover, the increments were also associated with fewer ventilator-free days. Flori also suggested that fluid overload itself may be a risk factor for mortality regardless of initial presenting severity of illness [2]. In another study involving 778 patients with septic shock post resuscitation also found that fluid overload increased up to twice the mortality rate [5]. Vincent et al. [7] in their research on sepsis patients found that each addition of a positive fluid balance after 72 h was associated with an increased odds ratio of mortality by 10%. Sutawan et al. [6] study also found that fluid overload was associated with mortality (OR 11.5; 95% CI: 3.7–35.6; p < 0.001) with a range of 12.9 ± 7.9% on 120 subjects.

2. Pathophysiology and measuring fluid overload

In general, the vascular endothelial allows free exchange of water, electrolyte, glucose, and nutrients components into and out of the tissue independently because of their permeability to the components. This transcapillary component exchange capability is affected by factors such as hydrostatic pressure, endothelial tone, and oncotic pressure. The fluid passing through the intact endothelial barrier and going to the extravascular generally will be reabsorbed by the lymphatic system to reduce edema. However, damage of endothelial barrier caused by the inflammatory process and edema will be easier to occur. The endothelial barrier is commonly known as glycocalyx, a network-rich carbohydrate and protein bond that regulates the process of exchanging fluid to extravascular (**Figure 1**) [8].

Beside its own endothelial tissue structure, intravascular volume stability is also regulated by baroreceptors located in the carotid, atrial, and afferent renal arterioles. The renin-angiotensin-aldosterone system (RAAS) will be readily activated resulting in natriuretic peptide secretion in the event of intravascular volume changes [10]. Activation of the RAAS system and the secretion of natriuretic peptides make water and sodium retained by the kidneys to maintain intravascular volume. Imbalance between intravascular and extravascular fluid or component like natrium will facilitate intravascular fluid to the interstitial so that edema, ascites, pleural effusion may occur. Some studies use FO percentage (FO%) as a tool to estimate the amount of fluid retention [9, 10].

$$FO\% = [(\text{fluid administrated} - \text{fluid eliminated}/\text{body weight when first arrived}] \times 100 \quad (1)$$

The fluids are measured in liters while the body weight measured in kilogram. FO% ≥ 10% is associated with high morbidity rates, such as worsening oxygenation levels, longer mechanic ventilator usage time, increased risk of renal replacement therapy (RRT), even to an increase

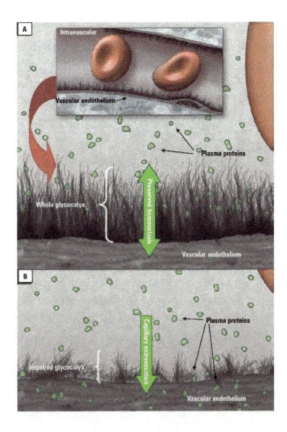

Figure 1. Schematic representation of glycocalyx [8].

in mortality. Patients who received RRT increased by 25% in critically ill patients. One of the risk factors is an increase in FO% levels between 10 and 20% [1, 11]. Similarly, in patients with ARDS, it is known that fluid retention increases mortality. Fluid overload with edema and extravasation manifestations into the third cavity is associated with failure of several systems such as the cardiovascular system, central nervous system, hepatic system, and digestive systems that stimulate malabsorption of nutrients and malnutrition in children. Fluid management for each critical illness in children is not the same depending on the clinical condition of the patient, but patients with high levels of FO% more frequently can cause failure of several organs [1–3, 12].

3. Pathophysiology fluid overload in sepsis and ARDS

In ARDS patients, some theories suggest that fluid overload can aggravate the patient's condition. Widespread injury of both lung and systemic endothelium with a resultant increase in permeability and expression of adhesion molecule is characteristic of ARDS/ALI [13]. Injury to the microvascular endothelium of the lung was first known almost 30 years ago [14, 15]. A variety of circulating markers of endothelial cell injury and activation have been studied in patients with ARDS/ALI. Endothelin-1, a vasoconstrictor and proinflammatory peptide is released by endothelial cell as a result of injury, is increased in the plasma of patients with ARDS/ALI as is von Willebrand factor (VWF) antigen, another marker of endothelial cell activation and injury [13, 16]. Higher levels of plasma VWF were independently associated with mortality by multivariate analysis in two independent studies. Although injury to the lung microvascular endothelial is the underlying cause of increased permeability pulmonary edema in ARDS/ALI, endothelial injury and activation may also lead to obstruction or destruction of the lung microvascular bed in ARDS/ALI case [15]. The degree of obstruction and destruction of the lung microvascular bed is an important determinant of outcome and can be estimated by the pulmonary dead space fraction [1, 15].

Fluid management in sepsis patients is necessary to increase the perfusion of vital organs in order to restore the patient's hemodynamics. However, there has been no research suggesting the amount of fluid dosage in sepsis patients. Based on early goal directed therapy (EGDT) for the treatment of severe sepsis and septic shock, targeted fluid therapy used central venous pressure (CVP) [7, 17]. However, the target cvp is 8–12 mmHg to ensure intravascular volume. However, the EGDT guidelines do not limit the extent to which these fluids should be administered to patients. Even some recent studies suggest that fluid administration according to the EGDT concept has been abandoned because it is more likely to make hypervolemia and increase mortality rates in the first 48, 72, and 96 h post-EGDT [17]. This increase in mortality rates is more likely to be caused by FO, as FO may aggravate capillary leakage and contribute to or worsen edema in patients' lung with sepsis and septic shock. FO can also create intraabdominal hypertension, leading to organ hypoperfusion that will eventually fall on organ failure [18].

4. Managing fluid overload

4.1. Composition of resuscitation fluids

There is no ideal fluid used for resuscitation of shock patients. At least the fluid used has a similar chemical composition to the plasma and can eliminate shock signals without adding fluid extravasation to the interstitial cavity. Currently, the fluid used is colloidal fluid and crystalloid fluid [19].

Crystalloids are more recommended as first-line therapy to restore hemodynamics in patients with shock [20]. Crystalloids are made up of ions with various tonicities and can be freely distributed. The saline liquor is more isotonic to the plasma but has a higher concentration of chloride and is more at risk of hyperchloremic metabolic acidosis and increases the risk of kidney failure [18]. The fluid such as the rringer is more hypotonic than the extracellular fluid and is also associated with hyperchloremia but has a pH that is more similar to plasma pH [19–21].

Colloid is a fluid containing macromolecules with the usefulness of increasing the oncotic pressure and maintaining the amount of fluid that already exists in the vascular and even absorb fluid in extracellular to intracellular [5, 8]. Colloids are classified according to natural (albumin) and artificial (gelatin, dextran, and hydroxyethyl starch (HES)) [7]. In contrast to the crystalloid fluid distributed among compartments, the colloidal fluid will remain in the vascular cavity for more than 16 h [8].

Gelatins, a polypeptide derived from collagen bovine, have the same extravascular extension as albumin but are associated with the risk of renal damage. HES is a high-molecular weight synthetic polymer and is associated with high incidence of renal failure and coagulation disease [8].

A study comparing the effects of crystalloid with HES found that the use of HES could reduce the amount of fluid intake (30% less than crystalloid), increasing CVP faster, decreasing the incidence of shock but increasing chances for RRT and increasing mortality [22].

4.2. Volume resuscitation

The resuscitation phase aims to restore intravascular volume, increase blood pressure, increase urine output, restore peripheral perfusion and increase consciousness level [17]. Aggressive fluid administration in this phase is associated with fluid overload [21]. The amount of fluid required in this phase also varies and depends on the individual patient [23]. Fluid management without adequate monitoring can increase the risk of volume overload [21]. Management using a vasopressor need not be delayed and aims to restore and maintain renal perfusion, optimize diuresis, and prevent fluid accumulation [10].

Predicting fluid delivery can reduce the risk of over-giving and unnecessary fluid [24]. Monitoring cardiac output and evaluation of vena cava diameter with ultrasound is one of the mechanisms used to monitor the amount of incoming fluid [25]. This method still has limitations due to the varied reference values that are used to assess the clinical patient, as each individual differs in the amount of fluid that enters depending on body weight, renal ability, and type of illness being suffered [26]. Some of these hemodynamic variables cannot be adequately calculated in patients with inadequate ventilation and receive low tidal volume. In the case of unstable hemodynamics, relative hypovolemia may occur due to the administration of sedative drugs or infectious processes [27].

Calculating central venous saturation and CVP does not show high sensitivity and specificity to predict fluid response [21]. It is estimated that more than 50% of patients are admitted to the ICU because of sepsis and do not respond adequately to this volume test [28]. Signs of tissue hypoperfusion such as lactate and central venous saturation are generally used to evaluate the appropriate time to stop fluid resuscitation [29]. A retrospective study of 405 septic patients receiving therapy based on the central venous saturation target and mean arterial pressure (MAP) protocols indicated a high risk of FO and mortality [30]. However, regular evaluation of venous saturation to evaluate resuscitation responses is more commonly used and is associated with fluid overload [31].

4.3. Maintenance volume

In patients with critical illness and treated in the ICU, FO should be avoided [23]. Treatment of fluid administration depends on each individual in the resuscitation phase. As described earlier, FO is associated with high morbidity and mortality [28]. After returning blood pressure or on children returning heart rate is more valuable, the primary focus is adequate oxygen delivery to the tissue, which is directly related to cardiac output, hemoglobin concentration, and arterial saturation [32].

Conservative fluid management is associated with increased oxygen levels, decreased ventilator usage time, and decreased hospitalization. Patients treated in the ICU room on average will get fluid overload problems. Beside direct administration of fluids through venous access, these patients also receive fluids through drug administration and nutrient feeding and thus increasing the risk of fluid overload. However, in the maintenance phase, it is important to minimize the administration of unnecessary fluids [1, 33]. When FO is identified in a patient with stable hemodynamic and vasopressor reduction, fluid reduction should be the primary target to avoid negative FO effects [32].

4.4. How to monitor fluid overload in our patients?

Conventional indicators, such as MAP, pulse, weight, peripheral edema, are not reliably used in patients with critical illness. MAP and pulse rate are highly fluctuative due to drug use. Indicators of fluid volume such as end-diastolic volume and intrathoracic volume may be useful but still require further study for clinical validation. Cardiac index monitoring and ejection fractions can be used to diagnose FO. In patients with mechanical ventilation, the absence of variation in pulse pressure may indicate the presence of FO [10].

A study of 49 patients using Doppler crosslinks could predict better diuresis using the index compared with changes in pulse pressure and increased MAP after fluid administration. This suggests that renal hemodynamic enhancement is essential for the occurrence of urinary output and reduces FO [34].

In sepsis patient with hypotension, the renal autoregulation mechanism is damaged by microcirculation changes. In this phase, vasopressor administration is often used to keep renal perfusion adequate, and a diuretic process still exists. Research in adults who analyzed the use of noradrenaline to keep MAP between 65 and 75 mmHg showed increased renal perfusion, with increased urine output, and less likely to require RRT. Furthermore, noradrenaline administration in patients with septic shock becomes an option for optimizing renal perfusion. The target of MAP in patients with septic shock differs depending on the history of blood pressure in patients, and patients with a normal history of takanan do not show significant gains for achieving MAP targets [35].

The use of loop diuretics such as furosemide to prevent fluid retention was said effective for inducing diuresis in children and adults. Low doses of diuretics (furosemide = 0.2 mg/kg/dose) may prevent the acute episode from hypovolemia. Continuous administration of furosemide infusions (0.1–0.3 mg/kgbb/day) may also be performed, and both can maintain drug concentrations in the renal tubules and prevent compensatory mechanisms of sodium reabsorption. A decrease in blood volume is also avoided to avoid hemodynamic deterioration. The use of long diuretics can cause resistance and known to use combination of loop diuretic and thiazide are also said to be effective [23].

The use of sedation drugs may cause vasiness and increase hemodynamic instability and thus increases the risk of excessive fluid administration. Provision of sedation also makes the patient should bed rest and is a risk factor for microvascular dysfunction and eventually fluid fertilization returns. This of course increases the time of ventilator use and increases the length of stay in the ICU and the hospital [36].

5. Conclusion

Fluid overload is an event that is often found in the intensive care room of children. This is in because the more severe the patient the more fluid administered, not only through infusion, but the provision of drugs and nutrients are also no less. Some recent research has found that fluid overload has many negative effects, particularly, in patients who have both sepsis and ARDS. In sepsis and ARDS patients, the initial fluid administration is able to increase disease survival rate but at 48, 72 and 96 h of fluid administration may result in an increase in mortality. Strength monitoring and restriction of fluid volume after resuscitation phase become an important step in order not to fall on fluid overload. Resuscitation should be subjective, and when the hemodynamic is stable, the volume of fluid should be handled either by direct reduction or by diuretics. Fluid overload generally associated with increased mortality, morbidity, duration of mechanical ventilation, length of hospitalization and the need for renal replacement therapy (RRT).

Author details

Dyah Kanya Wati

Address all correspondence to: dyahpediatric@yahoo.com

Critical Care Medicine, Udayana University Sanglah Hospital, Denpasar, Bali, Indonesia

References

[1] Willson DF, Thomas NJ, Tamburro R, Truemper E, Truwit J, Conaway M, et al. The relationship of fluid administration to outcome in the pediatric calfactant in acute respiratory distress syndrome trial. Pediatric Critical Care Medicine. 2013;**14**:666-672

[2] Flori HR, Church G, Liu KD, Gildengorin G, Matthay M. Positive fluid balance is associated with higher mortality and prolonged mechanical ventilation in pediatric patients with acute lung injury. Critical Care Research and Practice. 2011;**2011**:854142

[3] Arikan AA, Zappittelli M, Goldstein SL, Naipaul A, Jefferson LS, Loftis LL. Fluid overload is associated with impaired oxygenation and morbidity in critically ill children. Pediatric Critical Care Medicine. 2012;**13**(3):253-258

[4] Sinitsky L, Walls D, Nadel S, Inwald DP. Fluid overload at 48 hours is associated with respiratory morbidity but not mortality in a general PICU: Retrospective cohort study. Pediatric Critical Care Medicine. 2015;**16**:205-209

[5] Semler MW, Rice TW. Sepsis resuscitation: Fluid choice and dose. Clinics in Chest Medicine. 2016;**37**(2):241-250. DOI: 10.1016/j.ccm.2016.01.007

[6] Sutawan RIB, Wati DK, Suparyatha IB. Association of fluid overload with mortality in pediatric intensive care. Critical Care and Shock. 2016;**19**(1):8-13

[7] Vincent JL et al. Sepsis in European intensive care units: Results of the SOAP study. Critical Care Medicine. 2006;**34**:344-353. PubMed: 16424713

[8] Aditianingsih D, George YW. Guiding principles of fluid and volume therapy. Best Practice & Research. Clinical Anaesthesiology. 2014;**28**(3):249-260

[9] Lopes CLS, Piva JP. Fluid overload in children undergoing mechanical ventilation. Revista Brasileira de Terapia Intensiva. 2017;**29**(3):346-353. DOI: 10.5935/0103-507X.20170045

[10] Subramanian S, Ziedalski TM. Oliguria, volume overload, Na^+ balance, and diuretics. Critical Care Clinics. 2005;**21**(2):291-303

[11] Ketharanathan N, McCulloch M, Wilson C, Rossouw B, Salie S, Ahrens J, et al. Fluid overload in a South African pediatric intensive care unit. Journal of Tropical Pediatrics. 2014;**60**(6):428-433

[12] Wang N, Jiang L, Zhu B, Wen Y, Xi XM, Beijing acute kidney injury trial (BAKIT) workgroup. Fluid balance and mortality in critically ill patients with acute kidney injury: A multicenter prospective epidemiological study. Critical Care. 2015;**19**:371

[13] Lorraine B. Pathophysiology of acute lung injury and the acute respiratory distress syndrome. Seminars in Respiratory and Critical Care Medicine. 2006;**27**(4)

[14] Alphonsus CS, Rodseth RN. The endothelial glycocalyx: A review of the vascular barrier. Anaesthesia. 2014;**69**(7):777-784

[15] Burke-Gaffney A, Evans TW. Lest we forget the endothelial glycocalyx in sepsis. Critical Care. 2012;**16**(2):121. DOI: 10.1186/cc11239

[16] Murphy LS, Wickersham N, McNeil JB, et al. Endothelial glycocalyx degradation is more severe in patients with non-pulmonary sepsis compared to pulmonary sepsis and associates with risk of ARDS and other organ dysfunction. Annals of Intensive Care. 2017;**7**:102. DOI: 10.1186/s13613-017-0325-y

[17] Zhang L, Zhu G, Han L, Fu P. Early goal-directed therapy in the management of severe sepsis or septic shock in adults: A meta-analysis of randomized controlled trials. (Research article) (Report). 2015;**13**:71

[18] Boyd JH, Forbes J, Nakada TA, et al. Fluid resuscitation in septic shock: A positive fluid balance and elevated central venous pressure are associated with increased mortality. Critical Care Medicine. 2011;**39**(2):259-265

[19] Raman S, Peters MJ. Fluid management in the critically ill child. Pediatric Nephrology. 2014;**29**(1):23-34

[20] Dellinger RP, Levy MM, Rhodes A, Annane D, Gerlach H, Opal SM, Sevransky JE, Sprung CL, Douglas IS, Jaeschke R, Osborn TM, Nunnally ME, Townsend SR, Reinhart K, Kleinpell RM, Angus DC, Deutschman CS, Machado FR, Rubenfeld GD, Webb SA, Beale RJ, Vincent JL, Moreno R, Surviving Sepsis Campaign Guidelines Committee Including the Pediatric Subgroup. Surviving sepsis campaign: International guidelines for management of severe sepsis and septic shock: 2012. Critical Care Medicine. 2013;**41**(2):580-637

[21] Ogbu OC, Murphy DJ, Martin GS. How to avoid fluid overload. Current Opinion in Critical Care. 2015;**21**(4):315-321

[22] Myburgh JA, Finfer S, Bellomo R, Billot L, Cass A, Gattas D, Glass P, Lipman J, Liu B, McArthur C, McGuinness S, Rajbhandari D, Taylor CB, Webb SA, CHEST Investigators; Australian and New Zealand Intensive Care Society Clinical Trials Group. Hydroxyethyl starch or saline for fluid resuscitation in intensive care. The New England Journal of Medicine. 2012;**367**(20):1901-1911. Erratum in Hydroxyethyl Starch or Saline for Fluid Resuscitation in Intensive Care. [The New England Journal of Medicine 2016]

[23] Ingelse SA, Wösten-van Asperen RM, Lemson J, Daams JG, Bem RA, van Woensel JB. Pediatric acute respiratory distress syndrome: Fluid management in the PICU. Frontiers in Pediatrics. 2016;**4**

[24] Carsetti A, Cecconi M, Rhodes A. Fluid bolus therapy: Monitoring and predicting fluid responsiveness. Current Opinion in Critical Care. 2015;**21**(5):388-394

[25] Marik PE, Monnet X, Teboul JL. Hemodynamic parameters to guide fluid therapy. Annals of Intensive Care. 2011;**1**(1):1

[26] Caille V, Jabot J, Belliard G, Charron C, Jardin F, Vieillard-Baron A. Hemodynamic effects of passive leg raising: An echocardiographic study in patients with shock. Intensive Care Medicine. 2008;**34**(7):1239-1245

[27] Walker LJ, Young PJ. Fluid administration, vasopressor use and patient outcomes in a group of high-risk cardiac surgical patients receiving postoperative goal-directed haemodynamic therapy: A pilot study. Anaesthesia and Intensive Care. 2015;**43**(5):617-627

[28] Joosten A, Alexander B, Cannesson M. Defining goals of resuscitation in the critically ill patient. Critical Care Clinics. 2015;**31**(1):113-132

[29] Rivers E, Nguyen B, Havstad S, Ressler J, Muzzin A, Knoblich B, Peterson E, Tomlanovich M, Early Goal-Directed Therapy Collaborative Group. Early goal-directed therapy in the treatment of severe sepsis and septic shock. The New England Journal of Medicine. 2001;**345**(19):1368-1377

[30] Kelm DJ, Perrin JT, Cartin-Ceba R, Gajic O, Schenck L, Kennedy CC. Fluid overload in patients with severe sepsis and septic shock treated with early goal-directed therapy is associated with increased acute need for fluidrelated medical interventions and hospital death. Shock. 2015;**43**(1):68-73

[31] Mouncey PR, Osborn TM, Power GS, Harrison DA, Sadique MZ, Grieve RD, Jahan R, Harvey SE, Bell D, Bion JF, Coats TJ, Singer M, Young JD, Rowan KM, ProMISe Trial Investigators. Trial of early, goal-directed resuscitation for septic shock. The New England Journal of Medicine. 2015;**372**(14):1301-1311

[32] Rewa O, Bagshaw SM. Principles of fluid management. Critical Care Clinics. 2015; **31**(4):785-801

[33] Grissom CK, Hirshberg EL, Dickerson JB, Brown SM, Lanspa MJ, Liu KD, Schoenfeld D, Tidswell M, Hite RD, Rock P, Miller RR 3rd, Morris AH, National Heart Lung and Blood Institute Acute Respiratory Distress Syndrome Clinical Trials Network. Fluid management with a simplified conservative protocol for the acute respiratory distress syndrome. Critical Care Medicine. 2015;**43**(2):288-295

[34] Moussa MD, Scolletta S, Fagnoul D, Pasquier P, Brasseur A, Taccone FS, et al. Effects of fluid administration on renal perfusion in critically ill patients. Critical Care. 2015;**19**:250

[35] Piva J, Alquati T, Garcia PC, Fiori H, Einloft P, Bruno F. Norepinephrine infusion increases urine output in children under sedative and analgesic infusion. Revista da Associação Médica Brasileira (1992). 2014;**60**(3):208-215

[36] Lunardi N, Bryant M, Smith K, Lowson S. Early mobilization in critically ill patients. ICU Director. 2012;**3**(1):17-20

Intra-Abdominal Pressure Monitoring

Zsolt Bodnar

Abstract

Pancreatitis, inflammatory processes or retroperitoneal haemorrhage, paralytic ileus, ascites, severe visceral oedema caused by extreme fluid replacement, blunt abdominal trauma, peritonitis, or even massive transfusion can be found among the triggering factors of intra-abdominal hypertension and abdominal compartment syndrome (ACS). The only possible way of establishing the diagnosis is to measure the intra-abdominal pressure (IAP), a widespread manner of which is the measurement through the bladder. In our works, we wanted to study whether the method of continuous intra-abdominal pressure monitoring is feasible within the everyday practice of diagnosing the conditions having increased intra-abdominal pressure. The globally accepted pressure measurement carried out through a urinary catheter and its classical so-called intermittent form has been employed worldwide in the intensive care units and surgical wards. The procedure is simple, yet time consuming, and the catheter connections and disconnections are sources of infection. The measurement results provide information only on the individual pressure values of the predetermined measurement dates. In order to eliminate these weaknesses and for the safe and quick measurements, the classical technique was replaced by a completely new method: the continuous intra-abdominal pressure monitoring. In order to determine the objectivity of the continuous intra-abdominal pressure measurement technique, we carried out a validation study on surgical patients with normal and elevated intra-abdominal pressures. The pressure was determined by both methods in case of all patients. Significant difference could not be observed between the results of the intermittent and of the new technique. In this chapter, we want to discuss in detail of this validation study appointing the strong advantages of the new monitoring process. Measurement of the intra-abdominal pressure is essential in the differential diagnosis of acute abdominal pathologies. Pressure measurement through urinary catheters for the monitoring of the intra-abdominal pressure, especially its continuous variant, is an excellently applicable method. Introduction into the daily clinical routine is highly recommended.

Keywords: intra-abdominal pressure, intermittent intra-abdominal pressure measurement, continuous intra-abdominal pressure monitoring, intra-abdominal hypertension, abdominal compartment syndrome

1. Introduction

Human body is subdivided into smaller or larger units by well-defined compartments. The function of these compartments is to mechanically protect and separate from one another the organs or organ systems situated inside them. Distinctively separated spaces of our bodies are the different fascial compartments, the skull, the spinal canal, the orbit, the pericardium, and the thoracic and the abdominal cavities [1]. The elasticity of the tissues of the separating walls (bone, muscle, connective tissue) have a strong determinative effect on the tolerance for volume or pressure changes exerted on the organs, which can be found inside these compartments. Compartment syndrome in a wider sense defines those changes that occur in the given compartments due to the increased pressure (which apart from some lesser and/or greater fluctuations is constant under physiological circumstances) and to the decrease in local circulation developing in consequence of this. Detrimental effects of the increased pressure are widely known and precisely described in the medical literature [1–7]. Herniation syndromes occurring as a consequence of the increased intracranial pressure, the clinical appearance of pneumothorax and haemothorax caused by pathological accumulation of air or fluids inside the thoracic cavity, as well as the concept of pericardial tamponade are known by everybody. Although approaching these from this point of view is not routinish, yet no one questions that all the above cases represent a compartment syndrome occurring as a consequence of the increased pressure having been elevated due to certain specific reasons. Upon mentioning, associations are immediately made to fascial compartments; however, the term compartment syndrome means the clinical picture of the entirety of pathophysiological alterations developing in consequence of the increased pressure occurring within a closed space; and this is irrespective whether the separating compartment itself is formed by the skull, the thorax, the abdominal cavity, or a given fascial compartment. A common characteristic of these syndromes is the permanent and irreversible damage that may affect the organs, which can be found inside the given compartment if quick intervention cannot be provided. If vital organs are affected, these damages can be life-threatening or may even lead to death.

Abdominal compartment syndrome (ACS) was first described in relation to abdominal traumatic injuries, but its occurrence is not a bit scanty in the general surgical patient material, despite the fact that its aetiology is completely different [1, 2]. Kron [8] was the first who albeit did not use the term itself, yet described compartment syndrome in 1984. It was again Kron who routinely used abdominal pressure measurement through bladder catheterisation [8], which became widespread by 1989; however, the fundamentals of the method were described 100 years prior by Oderbrecht. Later on, several research groups developed the method [9–13]. The creation of abdominal compartment syndrome as technical term is associated with the work of Fietsam et al in 1989. The golden age of ACS has been launched by the two papers of Schein and Burch published in 1995 and 1996, respectively.

Pancreatitis, inflammatory processes or retroperitoneal bleeding, paralytic ileus, ascites, and severe visceral oedema caused by extreme fluid replenishment, blunt abdominal trauma, peritonitis, or even massive transfusion can be found among the triggering factors of ACS; i.e., all factors that may and can lead to a sudden increase in the intra-abdominal pressure

(IAP, 5–10 mmHg under physiological circumstances), to conditions of intra-abdominal hypertension (IAH, IAP ≥ 12 mmHg) associated with organ or multiple organs' failure, or without intervention to abdominal compartment syndrome (IAP ≥ 20 mmHg, which is associated with the failure of vital organs) [2, 7, 11, 12]. Despite the modern and quick diagnostics and the adequate surgical interventions performed in time, the mortality of ACS is extremely high (38–71%). It affects practically all vital organ systems such as cardiovascular, respiratory, urinary and central nervous systems, as well as the parenchymatous organs.

The only possible way of establishing the diagnosis is to measure the intra-abdominal pressure. A widespread manner of measurement is the method used through the bladder [8–11]. The fundamental principle of the method is the law which says that if pressure is exerted on the surface of a compartment predominantly containing some kind of fluid, then this pressure imposed upon the practically incompressible fluid will be transmitted unaltered to each and every point of the affected compartment. Consequently, the IAP and the intravesical pressure values are strictly identical. If the bladder is filled with 50 mL of physiological saline and the previously inserted catheter is closed, then the pressure predominating the bladder will be transmitted to the catheter and become easily measurable through a sterile needle inserted into the catheter. This procedure was simplified by the working group of Sugrue [11], who placed a 'T-element' into the catheter, which rendered unnecessary the closure and insertion of it, and also significantly reducing the prevalence of infections associated with this measurement. To surmount points of weakness (laboursome, intermittent), Balogh and his working group [13] developed and validated the method of continuous intra-abdominal pressure monitoring (CIAPM). Owing to their modifications, the procedure of vesical filling, catheter closure, and needle insertion was smoothed away ('Balogh-Sugrue technique').

Treatment of ACS is nearly always surgical decompression. Within the frame of prevention or in the case of individual ACS responding well to conservative methods, non-surgical solutions may also be possible (evacuation of the intraluminar content, removal of the space occupying process, improvement of the tolerance of the abdominal wall, optimal fluid therapy, optimisation of the systemic and regional circulation) [14–16]. Success is greatly influenced by the aetiology of the given case and by the general condition of the patient. If IAP > 20 mmHg (and/or APP < 50 mmHg, where APP = abdominal perfusion pressure) and new signs of organic dysfunction are occurring, then the ACS is not responding to the conservative method, and the possibility of surgical decompression should be carefully considered.

Surgical treatment for all cases of IAH/ACS is decompression laparotomy with temporary abdominal wall closure or open abdominal treatment. Following decompression, the problem cannot be regarded as solved, and the conservative method should be carried further on (adequate medication, optimal fluid therapy) along with the constant monitoring of IAP. APP above 60 mmHg and IAP under 12 mmHg mean the solution of the IAH. If APP > 60 mmHg and IAP > 12 mmHg, then the conservative method is still well founded, but the decompression or the revision of the previous decompression is necessary in case of APP < 60 mmHg.

In the past few decades, the consensus definitions were elaborated and following several modifications were published again in 2013, the diagnostic method was brought to perfection, the therapeutic possibilities were revolutionised and developed to a high-tech level; however, the puzzling out of the pathophysiology in its entire depth and as an integer is yet to be achieved [17, 18]. It is known that the basis of the phenomenon is the co-dependent chain reaction of several physiological processes triggered by the increased intra-abdominal pressure, but the exact mechanism still remains in obscurity [14, 15].

2. Aims

The main goal of this chapter was the description of the advantages and disadvantages of the different techniques for monitoring the intra-abdominal pressure. In our works, we wanted to study whether the method of continuous intra-abdominal pressure measurement is feasible within the everyday practice of diagnosing the conditions having increased the intra-abdominal pressure, as well as the ACS. Our aim was not only to validate this new technique but also to bring it to perfection as well.

3. Comparative study of the traditional and continuous intra-abdominal pressure measurement techniques

3.1. Patients of the comparative study of the intra-abdominal pressure measurement techniques

To carry on the comparative study of the intermittent (traditional) and continuous intra-abdominal pressure measurement techniques, 20 patients with acute pancreatitis were involved. The selection of the patients was based on a random nature.

3.2. Measurement methods

The intra-abdominal pressure was measured on every patient, in every 6 hours, by both the techniques. To avoid the technical errors, all of the measurements were carried out by the same person. Patients were included into the study following the preliminary oral information and signing of the informed consent forms, for which the patients had the right and possibility of withdrawal made at any time without providing any justification.

3.2.1. Traditional (intermittent) technique of intra-abdominal pressure measurement

Prior to our study, protocolised intra-abdominal pressure measurements were never performed at our hospital. Sporadic pressure determinations were performed in one or two clinical centres; however, routine measurements defined in protocols could nowhere be mentioned. In order to carry out the initial pressure measurements, we performed intermittent measurements following the Sugrue technique [8–11]. The patients wore a simple bladder catheter (Foley balloon catheter, 16Fr-20Fr, latex or silicone). During the measurement, the urine collection bag was removed and the bladder was filled with 50 mL of physiological saline through the lumen of the catheter. In the next step, the lumen of the catheter was connected to a set designed and used for the measurement of the central venous pressure (B. BRAUN Medifix® pressure measurement scale) with or without the insertion of a T-tap. The zero point of the scaled measurement tube was designated in the medioaxillary line corresponding to the anterior superior iliac crest. After waiting for 1–2 minutes, at the end of exhalation, the value of IAP could be read off the scale in units of cmH_2O. The values read off should be converted to mmHg (1 mmHg = 1.36 cm H_2O). When the measurement was completed, the system and the bladder catheter were disconnected and the latter was connected to a urine collection bag.

3.2.2. Continuous intra-abdominal pressure measurement

The technique of continuous intra-abdominal pressure measurement was known from the international literature [13]. With the aid of personal consultations with the Australian working group, which elaborated the procedure (Prof. Zsolt Balogh), we perfected and further developed it, and subsequent to the elaboration of the ward protocol and of further training lectures held for the specialist healthcare workers, we—being the only such institution to do so—introduced it to the everyday routine practice. Taking into consideration the nature of the intra-abdominal pressure being oscillatory even on a daily basis, we considered the use of the continuous intra-abdominal pressure measurement technique to be essential for the everyday routine, as well as during the design of the studies. For the measurements, we used 18 Fr standard three-way bladder catheters (LubriSilTM All-Silicone Foley catheter, C.R. Bard, Inc., Covington, GA, USA). The catheter and the urine collecting bag remained connected for all the time. In order to perform the pressure measurement, the so-called flushing port of the catheter was connected to the insertion of a transducer to a 24-hour bedside monitor. The connection of the flushing port and the transducer was effectuated with a triple tap. The collapse of the bladder was prevented with physiological saline continuously perfused with the speed of 4 mL/h. The zero point for the fixation of the transducer was established in the plane determined by the axillary median line and the anterior superior iliac crest. After the system was set to zero, the measured data were continuously recorded, in which data could be easily read off from the bedside monitor. The actual IAP value appeared directly in mmHg and required no further conversion. Pressure values were read off in every hour. The IAP mean value determined on a daily basis was calculated as the average of pressure values recorded in 24 hours [3, 4].

4. Statistical methods

Between the two methods correlation was expressed using the Lin's concordance correlation coefficient and Bland–Altman's 95% limits of agreement, overall and also stratified for measurement time. The concordance correlation coefficient evaluates agreement on a continuous measure obtained by two different methods.

The concordance correlation coefficient combines measures of both precision and accuracy to determine how far the observed data deviate from the line of perfect concordance (i.e., the line at 45° on a square scatterplot). The coefficient increases in value as a function of:

- The nearness of the data's reduced major axis to the line of perfect concordance (the accuracy of the data).

- The tightness of the data about its reduced major axis (the precision of the data).

With all coefficient estimates exceeding 0.97 and immensely significant, the findings indicate a very high level of concordance between CIAPM and the intermittent method. Bland–Altman's 95% limits of agreement estimates are within the clinically non-significant ranges of ±2 mmHg.

5. Results

In order to determine the objectivity of the continuous intra-abdominal pressure measurement, we carried out measurements in patients with normal and elevated intra-abdominal pressures. Significant difference could not be observed between the results of the intermittent measurements and of the new technique. According to the statistical analysis, the concordance correlation coefficient was higher than 0.97 in all cases, which shows a strongly significant agreement between the two different techniques (**Figures 1–4**). The 95% limits of agreement of the Bland–Altman method were between the non-significant ±2 mmHg ranges (**Figures 5–8**).

According to our results, we can summarise that the continuous intra-abdominal pressure monitoring technique is a modern, safe, and accurate method for the IAP monitoring, which provides results immediately, in millimetre of mercury without the need of conversion.

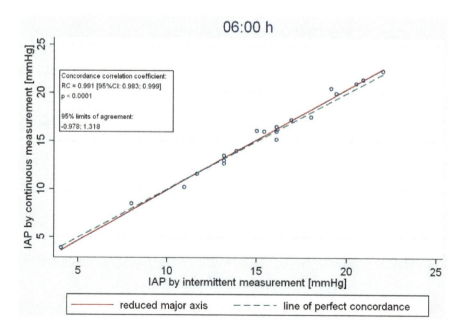

Figure 1. The concordance correlation coefficient was higher than 0.97 in all cases during the measurements carried out at 6.00 hour.

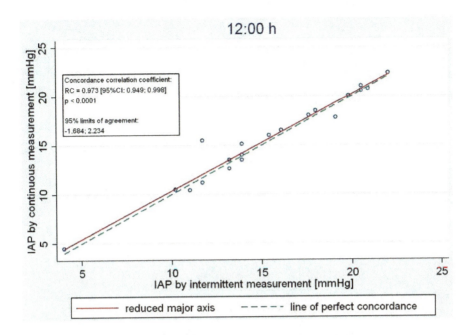

Figure 2. The concordance correlation coefficient was higher than 0.97 in all cases during the measurements carried out at 12.00 hour.

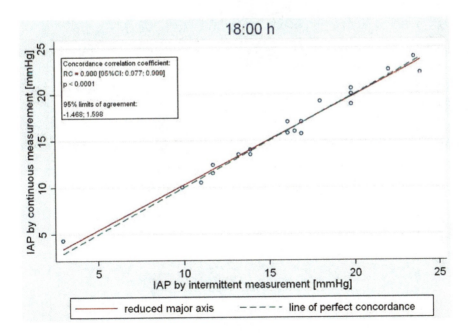

Figure 3. The concordance correlation coefficient was higher than 0.97 in all cases during the measurements carried out at 18.00 hour.

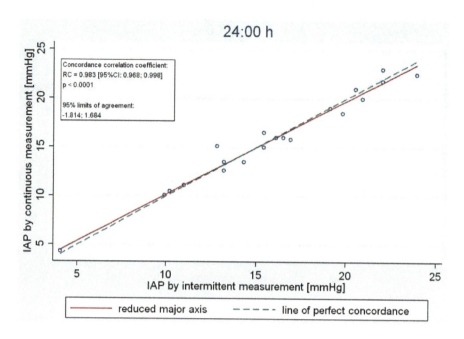

Figure 4. The concordance correlation coefficient was higher than 0.97 in all cases during the measurements carried out at 24.00 hour.

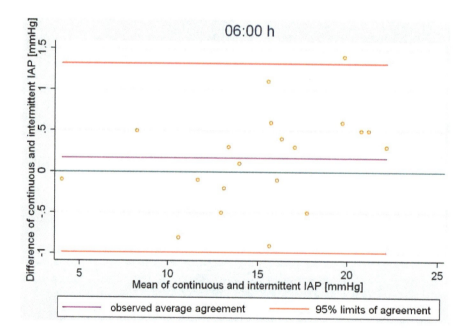

Figure 5. The 95% limits of agreement of the Bland–Altman method were between the non-significant ±2 mmHg ranges in all cases during the measurements carried out at 6.00 hour.

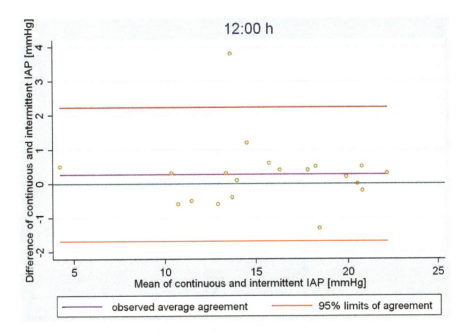

Figure 6. The 95% limits of agreement of the Bland–Altman method were between the non-significant ±2 mmHg ranges in all cases during the measurements carried out at 12.00 hour.

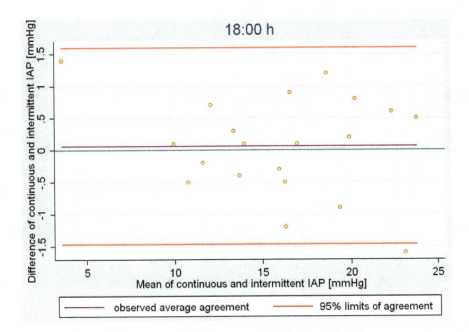

Figure 7. The 95% limits of agreement of the Bland–Altman method were between the non-significant ±2 mmHg ranges in all cases during the measurements carried out at 18.00 hour.

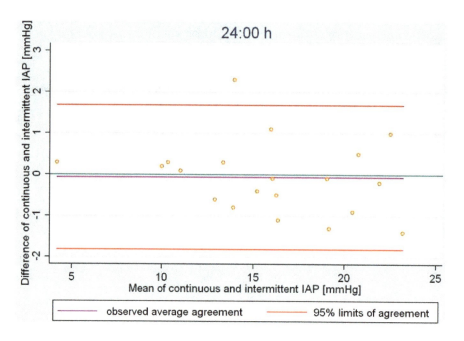

Figure 8. The 95% limits of agreement of the Bland–Altman method were between the non-significant ±2 mmHg ranges in all cases during the measurements carried out at 24.00 hour.

6. Discussion

Measurement of the intra-abdominal pressure is essential in the differentiated diagnostics of acute abdominal pathologies, in the following of surgery patients being in critical condition, in the prevention of the IAH/ACS, as well as in the monitoring of the already developed syndrome [3–5, 7–13]. The IAP (being within the normal range or increased) is never a constant value but has an oscillatory nature even less than 24 hours [12]. This nature was the main demand to develop a continuous control providing measurement method. The continuous intra-abdominal pressure monitoring technique was first published by Balogh and his working team in 2004 [13]. In order to determine the objectivity of the continuous technique, we carried out measurements in 20 patients, and we verified that the intermittent and continuous measurements are trusted methods of intra-abdominal pressure monitoring without significant differences between them. Following its first construction, the system of CIAPM can be operated without interruption until the next replacement of the bladder catheter (about 7–10 days), thereby eliminating the risk of infection originating from the catheter replacements in the intermittent measurements, as well as the need for extra work and tools.

Summing it up, the continuous intra-abdominal pressure measurement is the "gold standard" of the intra-abdominal pressure monitoring.

Pressure measurement through vesical catheters for the monitoring of the IAP, especially its continuous variant, is an excellent applicable method. Introduction into the daily clinical routine is recommended.

Author details

Zsolt Bodnar

Address all correspondence to: drbozsolt@gmail.com

Letterkenny University Hospital, Letterkenny, Ireland

References

[1] Balogh Zs, Butcher NE. Compartment syndromes from head to toe. Critical Care Medicine. 2010;**38**:445-451

[2] Bodnár Zs, Sipka S, Hajdu Z. The abdominal compartment syndrome (ACS) in general surgery. Hepato-Gastroenterology. 2008;**55**:2033-2038

[3] Bodnár Zs, Ary F, Bulyovszky I, et al. Continuous intra-abdominal pressure measurement technique (CIAP). European Journal of Anaesthesiology. 2006;**23**(Suppl. 37):197

[4] Bodnár Zs, Sipka S, Szentkereszty Z, et al. The gold standard technique for intra-abdominal pressure monitoring in septic patients: Continuous intra-abdominal pressure monitoring (CIAPM). Inflammation Research. 2007;**56**(Suppl. 2):213-214

[5] Bodnár Zs. Intra-abdominal pressure measurement. In: Orvostechnika és monitorozás. 1st ed. Boros: Szegedi Tudományegyetem ÁOK Szeged; 2007. p. 53

[6] Kirkpatrick AW, Roberts DJ, De Waele J, et al. Intra-abdominal hypertension and the abdominal compartment syndrome: Updated consensus definitions and clinical practice guidelines from the World Society of the Abdominal Compartment Syndrome. Intensive Care Medicine. 2013;**39**(7):1190-1206

[7] Ivatury RR. Pressure, perfusion, and compartments: Challenges for the acute care surgeon. The Journal of Trauma and Acute Care Surgery. 2014;**76**(6):1341-1348

[8] Kron IL, Harman PK, Nolan SP. The measurement of intra-abdominal pressures a criterion for abdominal re-exploration. Annals of Surgery. 1984;**199**:28-30

[9] Iberti TJ, Lieber CE, Benjamin E. Determination of intra-abdominal pressure using a transurethral bladder catheter: Clinical validation of the technique. Anesthesiology. 1989;**70**:47-50

[10] Iberti TJ, Kelly KM, Gentili DR, et al. A simple technique to accurately determine intra-abdominal pressure. Critical Care Medicine. 1987;**15**:1140-1142

[11] Sugrue M. Intra-abdominal pressure. Clinical Intensive Care. 1995;**6**:76-79

[12] Malbrain MLNG. Abdominal pressure in the critically ill: Measurement and clinical relevance. Intensive Care Medicine. 1999;**25**:1453-1458

[13] Balogh Zs, Jones F, D'Amours S, et al. Continuous intra-abdominal pressure measurement technique. The American Journal of Surgery. 2004;**188**:679-684

[14] Bodnár Zs, Keresztes T, Kovács I, et al. Increased serum adenosine and interleukin 10 levels as new laboratory markers of increased intra-abdominal pressure. Langenbeck's Archives of Surgery. 2010;**395**:969-972

[15] Bodnár Zs, Szentkereszty Z, Hajdu Z, et al. Beneficial effects of theophylline infusions in surgical patients with intra-abdominal hypertension. Langenbeck's Archives of Surgery. 2011;**396**:793-800

[16] Bodnár Zs, Sipka S, Tidrenczel E, et al. Ten years experience in abdominal compartment syndrome research 2004-2014. Orvosi Hetilap. 2014;**155**(44):1761-1770

[17] Malbrain MLNG, Cheatham ML, Kirkpatrick A, et al. Results from the International Conference of experts on intra-abdominal hypertension and abdominal compartment syndrome. I. Definitions. Intensive Care Medicine. 2006;**32**:1722-1732

[18] Cheatham ML, Malbrain MLNG, Kirkpatrick A, et al. Results from the International Conference of experts on intra-abdominal hypertension and abdominal compartment syndrome. II. Recommendations. Intensive Care Medicine. 2007;**33**:951-962

Endotracheal Intubation in Children: Practice Recommendations, Insights, and Future Directions

Maribel Ibarra-Sarlat, Eduardo Terrones-Vargas,
Lizett Romero-Espinoza,
Graciela Castañeda-Muciño,
Alejandro Herrera-Landero and
Juan Carlos Núñez-Enríquez

Abstract

Management of airway is mandatory in a critically ill child with severe trauma or any other situation that threatens his or her life. It is important, that clinicians who attend critically ill pediatric patients requiring airway management know the rapid sequence intubation (RSI) procedure, identify a patient with difficult airway, know the devices and techniques for the management of difficult airway, and look for receiving a formal training in endotracheal intubation (ETI). Future strategies for teaching and/or training clinicians in pediatric and neonatal ETI should be evaluated through conducting controlled clinical trials to identify which type will be the most effective by considering the less number of attempts and complications.

Keywords: endotracheal intubation, children, review, training, procedure

1. Introduction

Management and securing permeability of airway are mandatory in a critically ill child with severe trauma or any other situation that threatens his or her life. Airway's management can be defined as the performance of maneuvers and the use of devices that enable a correct and safe ventilation to patients that need this care.

Endotracheal intubation (ETI) is one of the procedures that every physician attending critically ill pediatric patients must not only know but also getting the skills and experience necessaries to effectively perform.

In this chapter, we will summarize the most practical recommendations of ETI technique in children. In addition, we will discuss important anatomical particularities of the children's airway. We include a section of devices that could help permeate the airway of pediatric patients with a difficult airway; and recent results of studies conducted regarding the association between the level of previous training in pediatric ETI and success rates.

1.1. Indications of ETI in children

1. Patient with an unstable airway. In this category, integrity of airway is affected by different infectious, anatomical and neurological diseases. Some examples are: (a) upper airway infectious (CROUP, bacterial tracheitis, etc.), (b) traumatisms, (c) congenital syndromes accompanied with macroglossia or micrognathia, (d) cystic hygroma, (e) branchial cleft cyst, (f) thyroglossal duct cyst, and (g) those patients with a large anterior mediastinal mass (non-Hodgkin lymphoma, acute leukemia, etc.). During childhood, the most common cause is infections [1].

2. Patient with neurological dysfunction secondary to trauma, seizures, metabolic disease, or toxic ingestion. Classically, we can find patients with a Glasgow Coma Scale (GCS) score of 8 or less, or a deterioration in the GCS score from 14 to 10.

3. Patient with impaired gas exchange:

    a. Hypoxia. One of the most common indications of ETI. Clinically, the patient presents with respiratory distress, tachypnea, increased work of breathing, and an increase in alveolar-arterial gradient. Some causes of hypoxia are airway obstruction, hypoventilation, ventilation/perfusion mismatch, hemoglobinopathies, abnormal pulmonary diffusion, and intracardiac right to left shunt.

    b. Hypercarbia. The pathophysiologic phenomenon consists of alteration in ventilation. There exists a reduced lung compliance and a V/Q mismatch increasing physiologic dead space. Alteration in ventilation can also be secondary to muscle weakness, altered mental status, exposure to toxins, or iatrogenic oversedation.

4. Patient with lower airway obstruction. Hypercarbia, tachypnea, increased work of breathing, wheezing, and a prolonged expiratory phase are characteristic. As lower obstruction progresses, dynamic hyperinflation and air trapping worsen, leading to a silent chest (inaudible breath sounds). This obstruction is common in asthma and bronchiolitis. We must remember that children can get intubated by this indication but it has been described an increase in mean airway pressure that may impede venous return. Therefore, under this indication children should only be intubated in EXTREME CIRCUMSTANCES [1].

5. Patient with a reduction of mechanical load, as seen in shock state and some patients with cardiovascular dysfunction.

2. Practice recommendations for pediatric endotracheal intubation

2.1. Rapid sequence intubation

By using rapid sequence intubation (RSI) method, a clinician can effectively achieve pediatric endotracheal intubation (ETI), however, we previously must identify if the patient has one or more of the following features related with a difficult airway [2]:

- To have congenital abnormalities related with a difficult airway such as Pierre Robins Syndrome and/or Treacher Collins Syndrome.
- A previous difficult ETI.
- A poor mouth opening, large tongue or tonsils, small chin, short mandible, decreased neck mobility, and/or an evidence of partial upper airway obstruction.

Note: later in this chapter, you can find information about the causes, techniques, and a variety of devices a clinician may use for the management of children with difficult airway.

2.1.1. Preparation

1. If it is not performed in an emergency setting (elective intubation), an informed consent must be obtained from the child's parents explaining the technique, complications, and benefits of performing the procedure [3].
2. All the materials to be used should be functional.
3. Team should consist of three persons (at least).
4. Patient's heart and respiratory rate, blood pressure, oxygen saturation, (capnography when available) must be monitored during the procedure.
5. Oxygen supply must be at least 10 l/min and suction equipment must be available and it must have pressures around 80–120 mm Hg.

Equipment

1. An appropriate mask and bag for ventilation. We must select the mask size that fits the nasal bridge and the chin of the patient without covering the eyes (**Figure 1**). Bag used for infants and young children is named pediatric bag (which provides a tidal volume of approximately 400–500 ml); for older children and adolescents, an adult bag should be used (providing a tidal volume of 1000 ml) [3–5].
2. Endotracheal tubes (ETs). Uncuffed ETs are mainly indicated for neonates, infants, and young children (<8 years). The correct size of these ETs can be calculated according to the equation (child's age/4) + 4. On the other hand, the formula (child's age/2) + 3.5 might be used for cuffed ETs. Other methods to calculate ETs size include comparing the child's fifth finger with the internal diameter of the ET or by using resuscitation tape such as the Broselow Luten tape, and it is recommendable to have one size larger and smaller of the selected tube.
3. Stylet. Adult sized for 5.5 tubes and beyond, pediatric ones for lower endotracheal tubes.

4. Laryngoscope handle and blade. The first one can be an adult or pediatric one, and the second can be straight or curved depending on the experience of the laryngoscopist. The blades used in pediatrics ranged from 00 (extremely premature neonates) to 4. Blades 0–1 are used for preterm and full-term neonates, size 1 for infants. At age 2, size 2 blade; at this age, a curved blade can be used. For ages 10 and above, a number 3 blade is recommended.

5. Colorimetric end tidal carbon dioxide devices or capnography monitors.

6. Tape or a commercial holder to secure the endotracheal tube.

7. Syringe for cuff inflation.

8. Nasogastric and orogastric tubes.

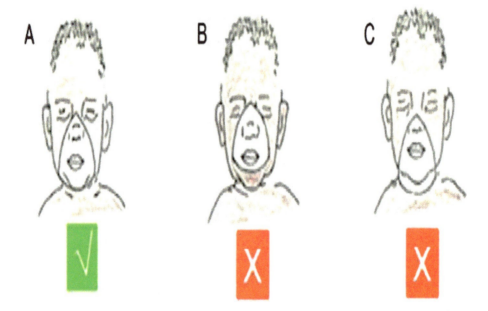

Figure 1. (A) The correct size for the child because it covers the area between nasal bridge and chin. (B) The mask elected is not correct, it covers part of the eyes of the patient. (C) The mask elected is not correct it covers the area far from the chin.

Tips and tricks

To remember all the preparatory equipment before starting intubation

You can use the **STOP MAID** mnemonic to remember all the preparatory equipment before starting ETI procedure:

Suction;

Tools for intubation;

Oxygen;

Positioning (sniffing position so that the external auditory canal is anterior to shoulder);

Monitors;

Assistant, Ambu bag with facemask, airway devices;

Intravenous access;

Drugs (sedation, neuromuscular blocking medications).

2.1.2. Preoxygenation phase

With all the necessary tools already prepared, next, we must position the patient for the denominated preoxygenation phase. This position consists in a sniffing situation avoiding hyperextension and/or hyperflexion of the neck. The correct sniffing position is the one with exterior auditory canal anterior to the shoulders (**Figure 2**).

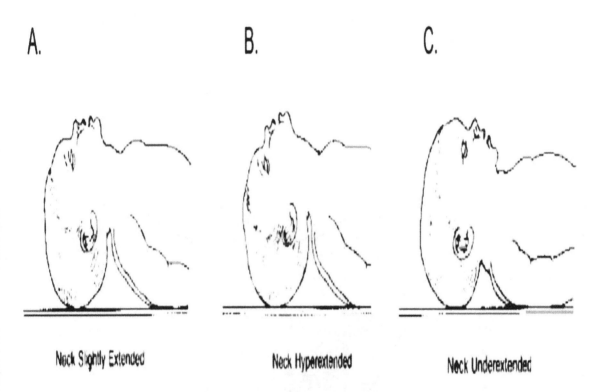

Figure 2. (A) Correct sniffing position is shown the external auditory canal is anterior to the shoulders of the patient. (B) Incorrect position because neck is hyperextended. (C) Incorrect position because patient's neck has hyperflexion.

Selection of ventilation technique relies on the number of persons available at preoxygenation phase:

- One-person ventilation technique. The head must be positioned backwards, using the C-E technique and the chin must be elevated pressing and sealing the mask to the face. Sealing is very important. We may corroborate that ventilation technique is correct when elevation of the chest is observed (**Figure 3**).

- Two-person ventilation technique. One member of the health care professional team will use the C-E technique but now with two hands while the other person will be pressing the bag (**Figure 4**).

After patient is positioned, then, ventilation must start with 100% inspired oxygen creating an oxygen reservoir. It is important to avoid hyperventilation. Therefore, a slow ventilation lasting around a second each must be applied being overall preoxygenation phase duration 3–5 min.

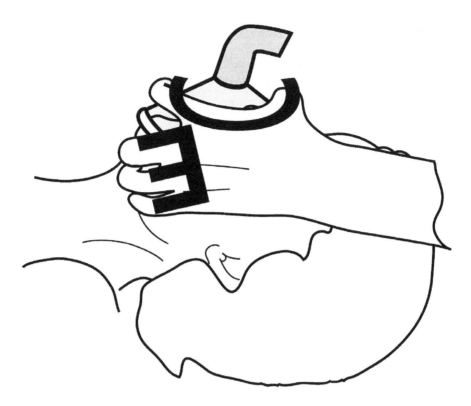

Figure 3. One-person C-E ventilation technique is illustrated.

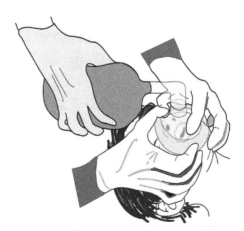

Figure 4. Two-person C-E ventilation technique. First person is doing a double hand C-E maneuver while a second person (not shown in the image) is pressing the bag.

2.1.3. Sedation and neuromuscular blockade

Premedication increases success rate of pediatric ETI independently from degree of previous training [6]. By using the rapid sequence intubation in children, success rate of 52% and a complication rate of 61% can be achieved [7], however, sedation can be omitted in obtunded or comatose patients and neuromuscular blockade must be avoided in patients with difficult airway. **Table 1** summarizes the drugs, indications, and doses used for sedation and neuromuscular blockade during pediatric ETI procedure.

Medications		Indications	Doses (IV)
Sedation	Etomidate	Hemodynamic instability, neuroprotective	0.3 mg/kg
	Ketamine	Hemodynamic instability, patients with bronchospasm and septic shock	1–2 mg/kg
	Midazolam	It can cause hemodynamic instability	0.2–0.3 mg/kg
	Propofol	In hemodynamically stable patients	1–1.5 mg/kg
	Thiopental	Neuroprotection	3–5 mg/kg
NM blockers	Rocuronium	For children in which succinylcholine is contraindicated	0.6–1.2 mg/kg
	Succinylcholine	Do not use in extensive crush injury, chronic myopathy	2 mg/kg

Table 1. Drugs, indications, doses for achieving sedation and neuromuscular (NM) blockade during pediatric ETI.

2.1.4. Procedure

Clinician may most easily perform direct laryngoscopy by standing behind to the patient's head and with height of the bed adjusted to the level of the laryngoscopist xiphoid appendix (**Figure 5**). After sedation and neuromuscular blocking, the clinician must perform a scissor maneuver to open mouth before laryngoscopy. Then, laryngoscope must be held in the left hand (regardless of dominance), inserting the blade in the right side of the patient's mouth along the base of the tongue following the contour of the pharynx, and sweeping the tongue to the left.

Once the tongue and soft tissues are retracted, clinician must recognize the following anatomic structures: epiglottis, arytenoid cartilage, and esophagus (**Figure 6**). After identifying epiglottis, this must be elevated exposing the vocal cords by handling laryngoscope at a 45° angle. Next step, endotracheal tube (ET) must be inserted into the trachea by holding it (with right hand) like a pencil (**Figure 7**).

ET insertion in airway must be confirmed by the observation chest wall rise and down with ventilations, auscultation of breath sounds in both axillae and not heard over stomach, and, to observe an adequate oxygen saturation (>90%). Radiographically, a correct position of the

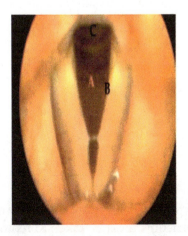
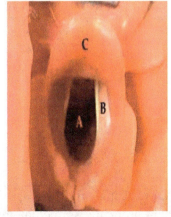

Figure 5. Proper position of laryngoscopist and correct introduction of laryngoscope after opening patient's mouth through a scissor maneuver (not shown).

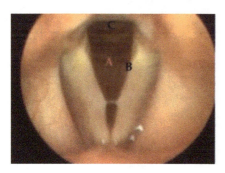 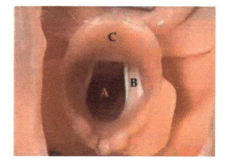

Figure 6. A comparison between a real larynx and a model. Structures of the larynx must be identified before trying to insert ET. (A) Glottis, (B) Vocal cords. (C) Epiglottis.

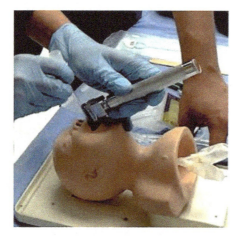

Figure 7. ET is introduced like a pencil into the airway.

Tips and tricks

To identify epiglottis and/or glottic structures

If epiglottis and/or glottic structures are not visible, blade must be pulled back slowly until they are visible. Other useful technique for helping to identify epiglottis and/or glottic structures is the named "Sellick maneuver" or so known as "cricoid pressure" (**Figure 8**). To perform it, another member of the reanimation team slightly push the region of cricoid cartilage while laryngoscopist observes the structures and introduce ET.

To calculate ETT length insertion

ET length insertion can be determined by any of the following two formulas [5, 8, 9]:

#1- (Patient's age (in years)/2) + 12

#2- ET internal diameter * 3

Note: we recommend first equation because it has been reported as more accurate.

---

tube is below the thoracic inlet and 3 cm above the carina (**Figure 9**). In case of ETT is located at esophagus or right bronchus, immediate measures must be taken to remove it and secure an adequate ventilation of patient (**Figures 9 and 10**).

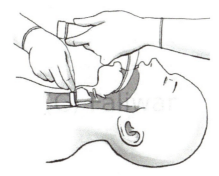

Figure 8. Sellick's Maneuver (also known as cricoid pressure).

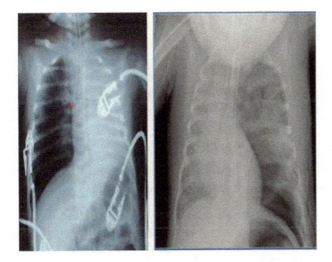

Figure 9. X-ray on the left shows a misplaced endotracheal tube which is in the right bronchus. Right X-ray shows a correct placement of the endotracheal tube, where the tip is located above the carina.

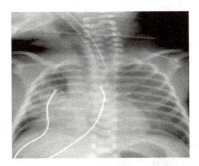

Figure 10. ET located in esophagus.

Tips and tricks [5, 10]
In case of acute respiratory deterioration after intubation
Remember the mnemonic DONE which can help you to identify the probable causes:
Deviation of ETT to the main bronchus or misplacement during suction. Signs that can suggest this are asymmetric elevation of the thorax or asymmetric auscultation, specially the right hemithorax.
Obstruction due to secretions obstructing tube's lumen.
Pneumothorax if are present signs as breath sounds diminished on the affected side, conduction of vocal vibrations to the surface of the chest may be increased, and hyperresonant at percussion.
Equipment, if problem is in the ventilator hardware or software.

3. Neonatal intubation

3.1. Indications

ETI in neonates can be most commonly performed as an emergency procedure or as part of an elective or semi-elective treatment:

1. Emergency. When mask ventilation or non-invasive mechanical ventilation fails, in case of structural or congenital airway abnormalities, diaphragmatic hernia, prolonged cardiopulmonary resuscitation, if thoracic compressions are needed, surfactant administration and for direct tracheal aspirations if thick secretions exist [11].

2. Elective/semi elective. Prematurity, positive pressure ventilation lasting more than 1-min, in case of ET must be changed, and in patients with an unstable airway [11].

3.2. Important anatomical considerations in neonates

In comparison to older children, adolescents and adults, anatomy of neonatal upper airway structures is different, being neonates a subpopulation where the ETI becomes a challenge. Some of these differences are the following: (a) a tongue proportionately larger, in consequence, trying to sweep it during ETI might be difficult and its backward movement might result in an airway obstruction; (b) epiglottis is longer, narrower, less flexible, and sometimes omega-shaped; (c) a cranial position of larynx can be an obstacle for observing the glottis during laryngoscopy, being this issue the reason why is preferable to use straight blades rather than curved ones in neonates; and (d) trachea is proportionally shorter and narrower [12, 13].

It is important to highlight, that neonates <1000 g, >4000 g, or those with congenital craniofacial abnormalities have less chance to be intubated at first attempt, representing a subgroup of neonates with a difficult airway which require special attention [14].

On the other hand, each attempt of intubation in neonates provokes injury of the mucosa which subsequently leads to an inflammation decreasing the caliber of the field of observation, and therefore, making the intubation less effective. Currently, it has been recommended a limit of 20 s for each intubation attempt in neonates, and if it fails, the ET must be removed and patient must be ventilated with a mask-bag reservoir until recovery [11, 15, 16].

Tips and tricks

Premedication phase in neonates is different from older children

In neonates, premedication phase must be only used as part of an elective ETI and not for emergency situations.

The American Academy of Pediatrics (AAP) and the Canadian Pediatric Society (CPS) recommend a combination of vagolytic agents and neuromuscular blockers for premedication phase in neonates. Also, the AAP recommends that muscular blockers and sedatives must not be used alone without analgesia [3].

Tips and tricks

ET size election for neonates

Election of ET size based on neonate's weight and gestational age:

Weight (g)	Gestational age (weeks)	ET size (internal diameter in mm)
<1000	<28	2.5
1000–2000	28–34	3.0
>2000	>34	3.4

3.3. Estimating length insertion of ET in neonates

Two methods may be used, and the objective is to place the tip of ET in the middle portion of trachea.

a. DNT method

   We must add 1 cm to the distance (cm) between the newborn's nasal septum and ear tragus (**Figure 11**) [17].

b. Gestational age method (**Table 2**)

c. "7-8-9 rule" method: in 1979, Tochen described a simple equation for the ET insertion length based on patient's weight at birth.

   Formula: $1.17 * \text{weight at birth (kg)} + 5.58$.

This equation has been supported by the AAP and the American Heart Association (AHA), establishing ET insertion length can be calculated by adding 6 cm to the newborn weight (e.g., for a newborn weighing 1 kg = 1 + 6 = 7 cm), from the patient's lip [14].

Tips and tricks

ET length insertion when nasotracheal intubation is used

When nasotracheal intubation is performed, the ET length must increase in 20% (e.g., for a newborn weighing 2 kg: (2 kg + 6) × 1.2 = 9.6 cm). We must also take in consideration that the 7-8-9 rule can overestimate the insertion length in newborns with a birth weight less than 1000 g. In consequence, it is preferred to use the gestational age method (**Table 2**) [18].

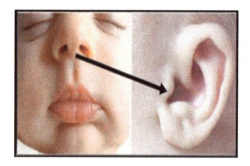

Figure 11. DNT method.

Gestational age (weeks)	ET length insertion (cm) from the patient's lips	Weight (g)
23–24	5.5	500–600
25–26	6.0	700–800
27–29	6.5	900–1000
30–32	7.0	1100–1400
33–34	7.5	1500–1800
35–37	8.0	1900–2400
38–40	8.5	2500–3100
41–43	9.0	3200–4200

Table 2. Gestational age method to calculate ET length insertion [18].

4. Management of the child with difficult airway (DA)

Difficult airway can be defined as the clinical situation in which a conventionally trained physician has trouble for achieving an effective upper airway ventilation with a face mask, for tracheal intubation or both and where interact patient's factors, setting conditions and operator skills [19]. First, we must evaluate child's airway to identify those clinical, and/or laboratory factors that could make difficult to achieve ETI. Among the anatomical factors related with DA are the form and size of mouth, nose, mandible, neck, existence of masses or congenital malformations, and other childhood diseases that eventually could difficult ETI (**Figure 12**, **Tables 3** and **4**) [20–24].

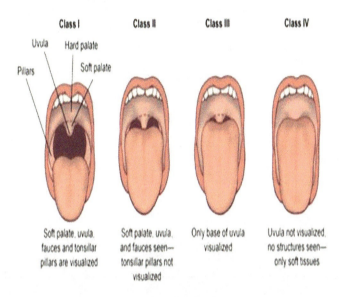

Figure 12. Difficult airway for ETI based on modified Mallampati classification [25, 26].

- Cranium's bone displacement. Apert syndrome, Crouzon syndrome, hydrocephalus
- Mandible hypoplasia. Pierre Robin syndrome, Treacher Collins syndrome, Goldenhar syndrome, Apert syndrome
- Abnormal neck mobility. Klippel-Fleil syndrome, Down syndrome, mucopolisacaridosis
- Limited oral aperture: Sheldon Freedman syndrome, Hallerman-Strieff syndrome, bullous epidermolysis
- Small oral cavity: Pierre Robin syndrome, Treacher-Collins syndrome
- Macroglossia: hypothyroidism, Beckwith Wiedemann syndrome, Down syndrome, mucopolisacaridosis
- Airway or neck masses: cystic hygroma, teratomas, hemangiomas
- Laryngeal or subglottic anomalies

Table 3. Pediatric syndromes associated with DA.

4.1. Devices and techniques for the management of the child with DA

DA devices can be classified according to the anatomical structure from where they will act and/or on their optical properties [27]:

4.2. Supraglottic airway devices

4.2.1. Classic laryngeal mask

It was developed in 1980 by Dr Archie Brain and forms part of the rescue devices in the ASA algorithm for the difficult airway management. It was designed to be situated in the

Infectious	Traumatic	Neoplastic	Inflammatory	Neurologic	Other
• Epiglottitis • Abscess (sub-mandibular, retropharyngeal, Ludwig's angina) • Croup • Papillomatosis	• Foreign body • Cervical column lesion • Skull base fracture • Maxillary or mandible lesion • Laryngeal fracture • Postintubation laryngeal edema • Facial trauma • Burns	• Upper airway tumors (pharynx, larynx) • Inferior airway tumors (trachea, bronchi, mediastinal) • Post-radiation area	• Angioedema • Anaphylactic shock (laryngeal edema) • Anquilosis • Juvenile Rheumatoid arthritis	• Spastic cerebral paralysis • Tetanus	• Lung hemorrhage • Obesity • Cranium-facial malformations • Micrognathia • Superior incisive protrusion • Short and wide neck • Big tongue • Previous intubation difficulty • Oral aperture limitation • Clift lip and palate • Mallampati classes 3 or 4 (**Figure 12**)

Table 4. Childhood diseases associated with DA.

hypopharynx, with an anterior aperture situated at the glottis entrance, the mask's border is made of a silicone inflatable cuff, sealing the hypopharynx permitting positive pressure ventilation (less than 20 cm H_2O). The mask is introduced using the index finger of the dominant hand as a guide towards the hypopharynx, following the palate's curvature, until a resistance is felt, then the cuff must be inflated with a determined volume (the specific volume comes in a legend on the mask itself and depends of the number of the mask). Choosing the size mask depends on the weight of the patient. As complications of the procedure we can find aspiration of gastric contents, uvula, and pharyngeal pillars lesions (**Figure 13**).

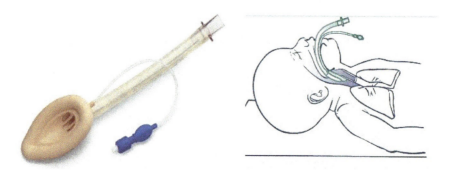

Figure 13. Laryngeal mask.

4.2.2. ProSeal laryngeal mask airway

In 2000 Brain published the description of a new laryngeal mask that tried to improve the airway's protection against gastric aspiration. This was accomplished by including a second tube lateral to the airway's tube and which in its distal end is located on the tip of the mask. This tube has the function of separating the digestive tract from the respiratory, and also Permits accessing the stomach with an orogastric probe (**Figure 14**) [28].

4.2.3. Fastrach or intubation laryngeal mask (ILMA)

This type of laryngeal mask is designed with the objective of achieving intubation through the mask itself, it consists of an anatomically curved rigid tube, wide enough to accept in it endotracheal tubes this end is united to rigid metal loop that makes the insertion much easier, removal, and adjustment of the position with one hand only. Once installed, and ventilation achieved an ET is inserted, the mask is then removed maintaining the tube in place, with a specially designed stylet, so that after the mask is removed the ET remains in place (**Figure 15**).

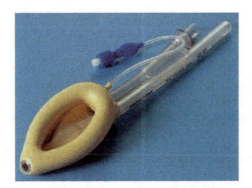

Figure 14. ProSeal laryngeal mask airway.

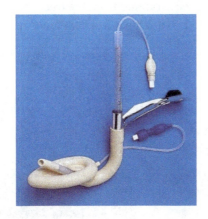

Figure 15. FASTRACH or intubation laryngeal mask (ILMA).

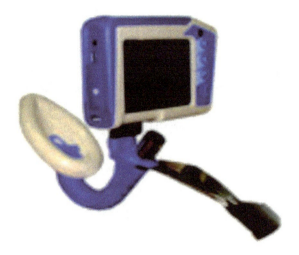

Figure 16. New type of Fastrach laryngeal mask.

Other type of *Fastrach laryngeal mask (2005) with an incorporated camera*, permits once it has been introduced into the hypopharynx, setting a monitor on the outer part of the mask so that it can be possible introducing an ET under direct vision (**Figure 16**).

4.2.4. Combitube

This device can only be used to ventilate in emergency situations. It was designed in Austria in the year 1980. Insertion is easy for any person and insertion is blindfold. It consists of a double lumen latex tube that combines the functions of an esophageal obturator and a conventional ET. Combitube has two balloons which inflate from the exterior. First one corresponds to an oropharyngeal balloon (85–100 ml of capacity) situated in a proximal position to the pharyngeal perforations with a function of serves as a sealing of the oral and nasal cavity; second one, is called traqueo-esophagic balloon, and needs a volume of 12–15 ml to seal the trachea or esophagus. Combitube can be placed either in the esophagus or in trachea, and in case of tube passes to the esophagus, the patient can still be ventilated because the perforations existing in combitube esophageal lumen, and the stomach can be aspirated from the tracheal lumen. In case of combitube is set in the trachea, the patient can also be ventilated from the trachea lumen (**Figure 17**) [29, 30].

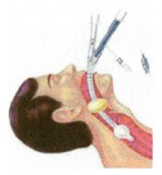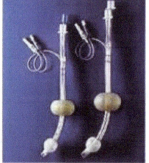

Figure 17. Combitube.

4.3. Transglottic airway devices

4.3.1. Gum Elastic Bougie

Eschman Guide or *Gum Elastic Bougie* (*GEB*) is a semi-flexible guide of polyester covered in resin (to avoid laryngeal trauma). GEB has a 15-Fr diameter and can be introduced in 6 mm internal diameter tubes. Insertion technique consists of sliding the angulated tip underneath the epiglottis, then, dragging at the tracheal cartilages must be perceived (**Figure 18**) [31].

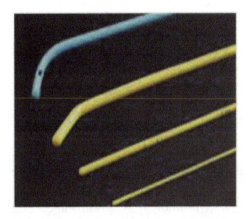

Figure 18. Gum Elastic Bougie (GEB).

4.3.2. Lightwand device (Trachlight)

In some countries, a lighted stylet is used for ETI, this is the called *Trachlight*. It is based on transillumination of the soft tissue of the neck with a high effectivity for achieving intubation in an approximate time of 25 s (**Figure 19**) [32].

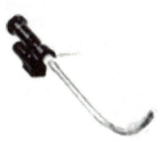

Figure 19. Lightwand device (Trachlight).

4.4. Optical devices

4.4.1. Video laryngoscopes

They are laryngoscopes that carry in its distal blade's end a high-resolution video camera to visualize the glottis and to introduce an ET without the need of observing the glottis directly but through a high-resolution screen which can be located in the same device or at the patient's side. Among the main complications reported are the soft palate lesions (**Figure 20**).

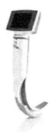

Figure 20. Video laryngoscope.

5. Insights and future directions

5.1. Direct laryngoscopy vs. video laryngoscopy

Learning curve (LC) in the case of the direct laryngoscopy requires of approximately of 45–50 previous intubations [33], while LC for video laryngoscopy is around 5 attempts. ETI using a video laryngoscopy is possible with little training, due to transmitted image from the blade's distal tip makes easier the visualization of the larynx entrance. When intubation attempts using Miller or Macintosh laryngoscopes or video laryngoscopy fail other methods to secure pediatric airway are recommended to be used (i.e. supraglottic devices). Recent studies have reported that ETI with video laryngoscopy even performed by less experienced medical personnel, increases significantly the success rate in the first attempt in comparison with direct laryngoscopy [34]; moreover, it has been reported that video laryngoscopy decreases the intubation time with less desaturation and less failure rate when it is compared with conventional laryngoscopy [35, 36]. Nevertheless, other video laryngoscope methods (GlideScope) implying other type of learning (mainly based on exploration), have resulted to be inferior to direct laryngoscopy regarding the time required for ETI [37].

5.2. Importance of formal training in pediatric ETI

Until date there is no standard definition for the term proficiency in pediatric/neonatal airway ETI. In a recent study, defined a formal training in pediatric airway management as having received at least 2 weeks of training by pediatric anesthesiology teachers. In that study was reported that after formal training, intubation success rate increased from 65.1 to 75.7% ($p = 0.01$), and it was observed a significant decreasing in the number of intubation attempts ($p = 0.01$). However, they did not find statistically significant differences in the time for achieving Intubation nor for the frequency of complications [38].

In a study conducted by Kerrey et al., where rapid sequence intubation technique was used, pediatricians in emergency departments and anesthesiologist had higher success rates (88–91%) in comparison to physicians in formation (45%) [7]. These results were similar to the reported by Goto et al. where intubation success was higher at the first attempt in pediatricians (OR 2.36; CI 95% 1.11–4.97) and in emergency room physicians (OR 3.2; CI 95% 1.78–5.83) in comparison to pediatric residents of the first and second year [39].

It has also been evaluated the skills for neonatal ETI between residents. Interestingly, skills significantly improved with a success rate from 27% during the first year of formation to 79% for the second year. Number of attempts also improved decreasing from 3.6 to 1.2 from the first to the second year, respectively [38]. This and other study results highlight the relevance of implementing training strategies from early stages of education in medicine to effectively achieve ETI in children with the less number of attempts and complications [6, 40, 41].

5.2.1. ETI training models, live models, and simulation training sessions for increasing success in pediatric and neonatal intubation

Recently, it has been mentioned that there are no differences in the learning curve or the skills for performing neonatal intubation by comparing live models versus ETI training models. Retention curves with a follow-up of 6, 18 and 52 weeks remain constant after 6 weeks and get lost after 18 and 52 weeks; although, retention is higher when skill levels are higher too [42, 43]. Additionally, it has been reported that educational interventions such as training sessions using didactic and simulation components have not been related with an improvement in intubation success rate; even, performance points decrease after 8 weeks of the intervention [44]. Importantly, other studies have not found differences in pediatric ETI success rate at first attempt by comparing groups with and without training [45].

6. Conclusions

It is important to highlight, that clinicians who attend critically ill pediatric patients requiring airway management know the rapid sequence intubation procedure, identify a patient with difficult airway, know the devices and techniques for the management of difficult airway, and look for receiving a formal training. Future strategies for teaching and/or training clinicians in pediatric and neonatal ETI should be evaluated through conducting controlled clinical trials to identify which type is the most effective by considering the less number of attempts and complications.

Author details

Maribel Ibarra-Sarlat[1], Eduardo Terrones-Vargas[2], Lizett Romero-Espinoza[3], Graciela Castañeda-Muciño[1], Alejandro Herrera-Landero[4] and Juan Carlos Núñez-Enríquez[1]*

*Address all correspondence to: jcarlos_nu@hotmail.com

1 UMAE Hospital de Pediatría Centro Médico Nacional Siglo XXI, Instituto Mexicano del Seguro Social, México City, Mexico

2 Unidad de Cuidados Intensivos Pediátricos, Hospital Infantil de México Federico Gómez, Secretaria de Salud, México City, Mexico

3 UMAE Hospital Gineco-Obstetricia No.3 "Dr. Victor Manuel Espinosa De Los Reyes Sánchez", Centro Médico Nacional La Raza, Mexico City, Mexico

4 Hospital de Traumatología y Ortopedia «Lomas Verdes», Instituto Mexicano del Seguro Social, State of Mexico, Mexico

References

[1] Rimensberger P. Pediatric and Neonatal Mechanical Ventilation. From Basics to Clinical Practice. 1st ed. New Delhi, India: Springer-Verlag Berlin Heidelberg; 2015. 1642 p

[2] Russo SG, Becke K. Expected difficult airway in children. Current Opinion in Anaesthesiology. 2015;**28**(3):321-326

[3] Emergency endotracheal intubation in children [database on the Internet]. UpToDate. 2015 [cited 2017-06-01]

[4] Staple L, O'Connell K. Pediatric rapid sequence intubation: An in-depth review. Pediatric Emergency Medicine Reports. 2013;**18**(1):1

[5] Kleinman ME, de Caen AR, Chameides L, Atkins DL, Berg RA, Berg MD, et al. Part 10: Pediatric basic and advanced life support: 2010 International Consensus on Cardiopulmonary Resuscitation and Emergency Cardiovascular Care Science with Treatment Recommendations. Circulation. 2010;**122**(16 Suppl 2):S466-S515

[6] Le CN, Garey DM, Leone TA, Goodmar JK, Rich W, Finer NN. Impact of premedication on neonatal intubations by pediatric and neonatal trainees. Journal of Perinatology. 2014;**34**(6):458-460

[7] Kerrey BT, Rinderknecht AS, Geis GL, Nigrovic LE, Mittiga MR. Rapid sequence intubation for pediatric emergency patients: Higher frequency of failed attempts and adverse effects found by video review. Annals of Emergency Medicine. 2012;**60**(3):251-259

[8] Curley MA, Arnold JH, Thompson JE, Fackler JC, Grant MJ, Fineman LD, et al. Clinical trial design—Effect of prone positioning on clinical outcomes in infants and children with acute respiratory distress syndrome. Journal of Critical Care. 2006;**21**(1):23-32; Discussion - 7

[9] Nichols D, Shaffner D. Rogers' Textbook of Pediatric Intensive Care. 5 ed. Philadelphia, PA: Wolters Kluwer Health; 2015

[10] Engorn B, Flerlage J. The Harriet Lane Handbook. 20 ed. Amsterdam; New York: Elsevier; 2014

[11] Weiner G, Zaichkin J. Textbook of Neonatal Resuscitation. 7 ed. Amsterdam; New York: American Academy of Pediatrics. American Heart Association; 2016

[12] Vijayasekaran S, Lioy J, Maschhoff K. Airway disorders of the fetus and neonate: An overview. Seminars in Fetal and Neonatal Medicine. 2016;**21**(4):220-229

[13] Murphy M, Walls R. Manual of Emergency Airway Management. 4 ed. Philadelphia, PA: Wolters Kluwer Health; 2012

[14] Johansen LC, Mupanemunda RH, Danha RF. Managing the newborn infant with a difficult airway. Infant. 2012;**8**(4):116-119

[15] Smereka J. Which laryngoscope method should inexperienced intubators use for child intubation? American Journal of Emergency Medicine. 2016;**34**(8):1729-1730

[16] O'Donnell CP, Kamlin CO, Davis PG, Morley CJ. Endotracheal intubation attempts during neonatal resuscitation: Success rates, duration, and adverse effects. Pediatrics. 2006;**117**(1):e16-e21

[17] Gray MM, Delaney H, Umoren R, Strandjord TP, Sawyer T. Accuracy of the nasal-tragus length measurement for correct endotracheal tube placement in a cohort of neonatal resuscitation simulators. Journal of perinatology. 2017:[Epub ahead of print]

[18] Kempley ST, Moreiras JW, Petrone FL. Endotracheal tube length for neonatal intubation. Resuscitation. 2008;**77**(3):369-373

[19] Auroy Y, Benhamou D, Pequignot F, Bovet M, Jougla E, Lienhart A. Mortality related to airway complications. Anaesthesia. 2009;**64**(4):366-370

[20] Cook TM, Woodall N, Frerk C. Major complications of airway management in the UK: Results of the Fourth National Audit Project of the Royal College of Anaesthetists and the Difficult Airway Society. Part 1: Anaesthesia. British Journal of Anaesthesia. 2011;**106**(5):617-631

[21] Adewale L. Anatomy and assessment of the pediatric airway. Paediatric Anaesthesia. 2009;**19**(Suppl 1):1-8

[22] Jenkins IA, Saunders M. Infections of the airway. Paediatric Anaesthesia. 2009;**19**(Suppl 1): 118-130

[23] Infosino A. Pediatric upper airway and congenital anomalies. Anesthesiology Clinics of North America. 2002;**20**(4):747-766

[24] Practice guidelines for management of the difficult airway. A report by the American Society of Anesthesiologists Task Force on Management of the Difficult Airway. Anesthesiology. 1993;**78**(3):597-602

[25] Samsoon GL, Young JR. Difficult tracheal intubation: A retrospective study. Anaesthesia. 1987;**42**(5):487-490

[26] Santos AP, Mathias LA, Gozzani JL, Watanabe M. Difficult intubation in children: Applicability of the Mallampati index. Revista Brasileira de Anestesiologia. 2011;**61**(2): 156-158 159-162, 184-187

[27] Miller DM. A proposed classification and scoring system for supraglottic sealing airways: A brief review. Anesthesia & Analgesia. 2004;**99**(5):1553-1559; Table of contents

[28] Brain AI, Verghese C, Strube PJ. The LMA 'ProSeal'–A laryngeal mask with an oesophageal vent. British Journal of Anaesthesia. 2000;**84**(5):650-654

[29] Agro F, Frass M, Benumof JL, Krafft P. Current status of the combitube: A review of the literature. Journal of Clinical Anesthesia. 2002;**14**(4):307-314

[30] Practice guidelines for management of the difficult airway: An updated report by the American Society of Anesthesiologists Task Force on Management of the Difficult Airway. Anesthesiology. 2003;**98**(5):1269-1277

[31] Viswanathan S, Campbell C, Wood DG, Riopelle JM, Naraghi M. The eschmann tracheal tube introducer. (Gum elastic bougie). Anesthesiology Review. 1992;**19**(6):29-34

[32] Inoue Y. Lightwand intubation can improve airway management. Canadian Journal of Anaesthesia. 2004;**51**(10):1052-1053

[33] Imashuku Y, Kojima A, Takahashi K, Kitagawa H. Endotracheal intubation training for clinical trainees in Japan is the anesthesiology training not necessary? Journal of Clinical Anesthesia. 2016;**31**:34

[34] Madziala M, Okruznik M, Cobo SA, Almira EF, Smereka J. Gold rules for pediatric endotracheal intubation. American Journal of Emergency Medicine. 2016;**34**(8):1711-1712

[35] Sakurai Y, Tamura M. Efficacy of the Airway Scope (Pentax-AWS) for training in pediatric intubation. Pediatrics International. 2015;**57**(2):217-221

[36] Moussa A, Luangxay Y, Tremblay S, Lavoie J, Aube G, Savoie E, et al. Videolaryngoscope for teaching neonatal endotracheal intubation: A randomized controlled trial. Pediatrics. 2016;**137**(3):e20152156

[37] Johnston LC, Auerbach M, Kappus L, Emerson B, Zigmont J, Sudikoff SN. Utilization of exploration-based learning and video-assisted learning to teach GlideScope videolaryngoscopy. Teaching and Learning in Medicine. 2014;**26**(3):285-291

[38] Leung SK, Cruz AT, Macias CG, Sirbaugh PE, Patel B. Improving pediatric emergency care by implementing an eligible learner Endotracheal Intubation Policy. Pediatric Emergency Care. 2016;**32**(4):205-209

[39] Goto T, Gibo K, Hagiwara Y, Okubo M, Brown DF, Brown CA 3rd, et al. Factors Associated with first-pass success in pediatric intubation in the emergency department. The Western Journal of Emergency Medicine. 2016;**17**(2):129-134

[40] Dongara AR, Modi JJ, Nimbalkar SM, Desai RG. Proficiency of residents and fellows in performing neonatal intubation. Indian Pediatrics. 2014;**51**(7):561-564

[41] Downes KJ, Narendran V, Meinzen-Derr J, McClanahan S, Akinbi HT. The lost art of intubation: Assessing opportunities for residents to perform neonatal intubation. Journal of Perinatology. 2012;**32**(12):927-932

[42] Andreatta PB, Dooley-Hash SL, Klotz JJ, Hauptman JG, Biddinger B, House JB. Retention curves for pediatric and neonatal intubation skills after simulation-based training. Pediatric Emergency Care. 2016;**32**(2):71-76

[43] Andreatta PB, Klotz JJ, Dooley-Hash SL, Hauptman JG, Biddinger B, House JB. Performance-based comparison of neonatal intubation training outcomes: Simulator and live animal. Advances in Neonatal Care. 2015;**15**(1):56-64

[44] Finan E, Bismilla Z, Campbell C, Leblanc V, Jefferies A, Whyte HE. Improved procedural performance following a simulation training session may not be transferable to the clinical environment. Journal of Perinatology. 2012;**32**(7):539-544

[45] Nishisaki A, Donoghue AJ, Colborn S, Watson C, Meyer A, Brown CA 3rd, et al. Effect of just-in-time simulation training on tracheal intubation procedure safety in the pediatric intensive care unit. Anesthesiology. 2010;**113**(1):214-223

Airway Management in ICU Settings

Nabil Abdelhamid Shallik, Mamdouh Almustafa,
Ahmed Zaghw and Abbas Moustafa

Abstract

Maintenance of patent airway, adequate ventilation, and pulmonary gas exchange is very important in critically ill patients. Airway management in intensive care patients differs significantly from routine surgical procedures in the operating room. The airway competence in intensive care unit (ICU) should be coping with the rapidly evolving advances in airway management. Therefore, efforts should be focused on the three pillars of airway master: airway providers as intensivists or critical care physicians, equipment, and operational plans. Not all institutions can afford all airway equipment in the market; however, they should make sure that critical care providers have a full access to the available tools and they are comfortable using it. Educational sessions and refresher courses should be tailored to meet the competence level of the ICU providers and equipment availability. Operational plan includes developing institutional airway protocols and implementing difficult airway guidelines. The protocols should consider different staffing models of ICU and make sure all the time at least one member of the team with the highest experience in airway should be always available. The aim of writing this chapter is to enable the intensivist to optimize their use of airway equipment and managing high-risk patients in ICU.

Keywords: tracheal intubation, videolaryngoscopy (VL), flexible fiberoptic intubation, bronchoscopy, percutaneous tracheostomy, extubation in ICU, high-flow nasal cannula (HFNC), virtual endoscopy (VE), airway ultrasound, supra-glottic airway devices, tube exchange

1. Tracheal intubation in ICU

1.1. Introduction

Tracheal intubation (TI) is one of daily practiced procedures in the intensive care unit (ICU), especially when the patient has respiratory failure or cardiovascular collapse. It involves highly skilled techniques that require much of training, practice, and expertise. The excellence in airway management in ICU is necessary for intensivist's every day practice, which when it is lacking does not only compromise the quality of care but also has a potential impact on patient safety.

The optimal intubation condition prevailing in surgical theaters differs a lot in nature than harsh and chaotic scenarios in ICU. The nature of those situations has three factors: the highly skilled anesthesiologists versus the intensivists; the compensated, well-controlled surgical patient versus the decompensated sick ICU patients; and equipment availability. That is why in ICU settings, the airway instrumentation-related complications have higher incidence than anesthesia settings. Among the contributory factors for high failure rates are the highly stressful environment, limited expertise level of the providers with different techniques of airway management, the physiological baseline for the patients, inadequate pre-oxygenation, unfamiliarity with new airway equipment, and the critical time factor in distressed situations in addition to the negative hemodynamic effects for the intubation medications.

2. Challenges in airway management in the critically ill patients

2.1. Response to pre-oxygenation

Effective pre-oxygenation is the first step for airway management. If it is done optimally by reaching PEO_2 of >90%, it extends the apnea safety time margin for critical ICU patients with already limited oxygen transport and when the intubation for airway control would be time consuming. The apnea time for oxy-hemoglobin to desaturate below 85% in postoperative period is 23 s in critically ill patients compared to 502 s in healthy adults [1].

The standard pre-oxygenation used in optimized surgical patients would fail to sustain adequate PaO_2 in critically ill patients with hyper-metabolic profile during apneic period for intubation.

The airway management encountered in a rapidly deteriorating patient with hypoxia from a life-threatening cardiopulmonary failure is not an uncommon daily ICU scenario. Lack of airway expertise is a high risk for multiple intubation attempts, airway trauma, esophageal intubation, and intubation failure, and consequences were adverse with high percentage of cardiac arrest or brain damage. Moreover, multiple traumatic trials by inexperienced provider could easily convert a simple airway to a difficult one due to airway edema.

2.2. Assessment and evaluation of the airway

Airway evaluation prior to tracheal intubation (TI) is the standard of care in anesthesia settings and should be routinely practiced in ICU before any TI. Many studies about airway evaluation in controlled anesthesia settings showed that combined airway tests are better than each test alone in terms of sensitivity and reliability.

Airway tests include Mallampati classification, thyromental distance, neck mobility, inter-incisor distance, and body mass index (BMI), which are all reliable predictors for difficult airway. Other scores include El Ganzouri test and LEMON test. El Ganzouri test is a numerical score, involves all the abovementioned tests: Mallampati classification, thyromental distance, neck mobility, inter-incisor distance, and BMI plus under-bite and previous difficult intubation history. LEMON test involves **L**ook Externally, **M**allampati class, **O**bstruction, and **N**eck mobility.

2.3. Drugs used for tracheal intubation, rapid sequence intubation

Hemodynamic changes during TI are predictable physiological consequences after airway management, which are attributed to three main factors: sympathetic system, cardiac contractility, and mechanical ventilation. Vaso-dilatory and cardio-depressive effects of medications, preexisting hypovolemia, and positive-pressure ventilation are major contributors to any predictable hemodynamic changes. Ketamine and Etomidate are anesthetic agents with a fast onset, short half-life, and tolerable hemodynamic changes. They are widely used in emergency settings to improve intubation conditions. Etomidate is an anesthetic agent with adrenal inhibition effect. A cardio-stable agent as Ketamine is preferable in ICU. The critical illness of ICU patients compromises the gastric emptying, making a rapid sequence intubation (RSI) a wise decision. Succinylcholine is a fast acting muscle relaxant with ultra short duration that is commonly used in emergency setting when there are no contraindications to its use. Muscle relaxants have its role in facilitating intubation; however, encountering cannot-ventilate-cannot-intubate (CVCI) scenario after giving muscle relaxants could lead to a fatal airway emergency. Studies found that physicians other than anesthesiologists are reluctant to use muscle relaxants before intubation in the ICU. A large data set found fewer complications, including in patients with difficult airways when muscle relaxants were used. In a prospective multicenter study, Jaber showed that tracheal intubation by muscle relaxants has less complications by 22 versus 37% when muscle relaxants were not used [2]. In another study in emergency department, Li et al. found a significant decrease in esophageal intubation with the use of muscle relaxants (3 vs. 18%) [3]. Succinylcholine should not be used in patients with hyperkalemia, congenital muscle disorders, and burn patients with difficult airway as it could lead to hyperkalemic cardiac arrest. As alternative to Succinylcholine, Rocuronium Bromide (1 mg/kg) can be used for rapid sequence intubation in critical care patients and can be reversed by Sugammadex Sodium.

2.4. Pre-oxygenation and tracheal tube confirmation

Pre-oxygenation before intubation is the standard of care. The standard pre-oxygenation used in optimized surgical patients could fail to sustain adequate PaO_2 in patients with respiratory failure. Randomized control trial (RCT) by Baillard et al. confirmed that pre-oxygenation done by noninvasive positive-pressure ventilation (NIPPV) prior to TI is superior to that done classically by a bag-valve mask device for a 3-min duration [2]. The patients who have been pre-oxygenated by NIPPV have higher pulse oximetric saturation (98 ± 2 vs. 93 ± 6%) and higher PaO_2 values during TI (203 vs. 97 mmHg) and up to 5 min into the post-intubation period compared with the bag-valve mask method. In acute respiratory failure,

NIPPV improves oxygenation by delivering high oxygen concentration, by unloading respiratory muscle, recruiting alveoli, and thereby increasing the functional residual capacity in such hypoxemic patients. To confirm the endotracheal tube placement after TI, classically chest inspection for bilateral equal expansion and chest auscultation for equal air entry on both sides have been routinely used. Recently, the American Society for Anesthesiology (ASA) has adopted end tidal CO_2 monitor as the standard of care inside the operating room. Confirmation of endotracheal intubation by capnography has 100% sensitivity and specificity. Continuous capnography waveform is recommended as well during chest compression for cardiac arrest victims [4]. Esophageal detector device is an alternative carbon dioxide-monitoring device. The endobronchial intubation must be ruled out by chest radiograph, as a part of post-intubation care.

2.5. Intubation "care bundle" management

Care bundles are the best evidence-based therapies that could guarantee the best outcomes when applied together than each therapy alone in the bundle. Intubation bundle has been developed to enhance the quality of intubation procedure by setting a package tool to be followed by any provider in any intubation scenario with every patient. This bundle focuses on standardization of the stepwise process and eliminating the individual preferences and technical variability. The bundle involves maintaining cardiovascular stability, gas exchange, and the neurological status while securing the airway. The proposed ICU intubation management protocol includes 10 elements bundle [2].

2.5.1. Pre-intubation

1. Presence of two persons.

2. (Normal saline 500 ml or colloid 250 ml) as fluid loading in the absence of cardiogenic causes of pulmonary edema.

3. Long-term sedation ready to start.

4. Pre-oxygenation for 3 min by NIPPV with the following parameters:

(FiO_2 100%, pressure support ventilation level of 5–15 cm H_2O, tidal volume of 6–8 ml/kg, and PEEP of 5 cm H_2O).

2.5.2. During intubation

5. Rapid sequence induction: Anesthetic medications include Etomidate 0.2–0.3 mg/kg or ketamine 1.5–3 mg/kg or Propofol-Ketamine mixture. Muscle relaxants include Succinylcholine 1–1.5 mg/kg or Rocuronium Bromide 1 mg/kg. Succinylcholine is contraindicated in the following condition, hyperkalemia, severe acidosis, acute or chronic neuromuscular disease, burn patient for more than 48 h and spinal cord trauma, otherwise Rocuronium Bromide is preferred.

6. Cricoid pressure or Sellick maneuver should be applied.

2.5.3. Post-intubation

7. Immediate confirmation of tube placement by capnography.

8. Nor-adrenaline infusion if diastolic blood pressure still low.

9. Start long-term sedation.

10. Initial "protective ventilation": Tidal volume 6–8 ml/kg of ideal body weight, PEEP 5 cm H_2O and respiratory rate between 10 and 20 cycles/min, FiO_2 100%, plateau pressure <30 cm H_2O.

Studies showed that the bundle lowered the life-threatening complications as severe desaturation, hypotension, or cardiac arrest by 21 versus 34%. Other moderate complications have lowered as well (9 vs. 21%) compared with the non-bundle group [2].

TI in emergency settings in unstable patients could lead to an acute airway emergency. The airway morbidity and mortality increase with unstable hemodynamics and failing oxygenation during emergency intubations. That is why tracheal intubation in the ICU may be life-saving or life threatening. Airway management in a deteriorating sick patient is a real ICU emergency which cannot be delayed. Rescue airway equipment as THRIVE, NIPPV, and tracheostomy should be ready as a backup when difficult airway is encountered. Fewer complications have been noticed when the TI was done by experienced providers. Familiarity with rescue airway techniques is helpful. The rhythm of ICU environment necessitates precise guidelines that are tailored to ICU settings. Hence, implementation of an intubation care bundle along with a pre-planned approach to difficult airway is essential for safe TI in the ICU.

2.6. Tracheal re-intubation

Particular issues as the need to re-intubate following a trial of extubation or accidental extubation are common in ICU. Re-intubation may be unexpectedly difficult in hypoxic, distressed, or uncooperative patients with multiple risk factors and in patients who have been extubated after prolonged intubation as airway edema is common sequela.

3. Videolaryngoscopy in ICU

3.1. Introduction

Videolaryngoscopy (VL) is an indirect visualization technique for the larynx mainly for the purpose of airway assessment or airway management especially in ICU area. The images from the video can be displayed, magnified, and recorded on a monitor. Video-assisted visualization has been evolved in airway practice after the pressing clinical need of difficult airway scenario and lack of new tools other than Macintosh/Miller blades. That was invented in 1940. After many years of clinical practice, the VL techniques have been approved by the American Society of Anesthesia (ASA) and incorporated in their difficult airway algorithms. VL is promoted as a first step to go in anticipated difficult airway scenario.

3.2. Indication or advantage over ordinary laryngoscopy

1. The first choice of elective oral or nasal intubation in adults, pediatrics, or neonates, in case of anticipated and unanticipated difficult laryngoscopy.

2. Reduces strain and stress of operator during intubation.

3. Diagnostic and recording of airway lesions, abnormal anatomy, and pathology.

4. Can be used for TEE probes [5], naso-gastric tube [6], double lumen bronchial tube [7], and throat-pack insertion.

5. VAFI techniques (video-assisted fiberoptic intubation).

6. Good teaching tool for junior staff.

7. Guide the assistant where to apply external laryngeal manipulation: BURP (Backward Upward Rightward Pressure).

8. Help presbyopic doctors especially in neonatal intubation.

9. Awake tracheal intubation [8] and in abnormal intubating position as lateral decubitus [9].

10. Less traumatic over ordinary laryngoscopy.

11. Reduce the cervical spine mobility in patients with unstable cervical spine or reduced spinal mobility [10].

3.3. Types of videolaryngoscopy (VL)

Many types have been introduced into the market, which has created many dilemmas for the practitioners which one to choose (**Table 1**). Each VL device is unique in its size, shape, and profile, which gives specific strength and weakness to each. As a dozen devices are being continuously added to the market, it would be challenging and impractical for the anesthesiologists to obtain and train on all of them. Ideal VL should be intuitive, lightweight, low profile, inexpensive, easily maneuverable, easy to learn and master, remote view screen, with memory storage capacity, and long-lasting rechargeable batteries. Special features are being added as antifog capabilities by heating of the lens. The device should be easily adaptable to different intubation techniques, for example, nasal and oral.

3.3.1. Video stylets

The rigid stylets were in practice for the last 25 years to facilitate retromolar intubation. The bending angle is 40° at the distal end with a view angle of 110°. The video RIFL has a rigid rod with a flexible tip to articulate till 135° by closing the lever by a handgrip.

The stylets are advocated when the mouth opening is limited; however, its applicability is restricted to oral intubation. The video stylets are bulky, requiring space in the room,

Rigid blades		Guided channels-Automatically shaped		Video stylets	
Standard blade	Angled blade	Channeled blade	Channeled airway	Rigid stylet	Rigid stylet + Flexing tip
Storz C-Mac	Coopdech VLP100	AirTraq	Total track (VLM) Video Laryngeal Mask	Bonfils	RIFL
	Storz DCI	Pentax AWS			Shikani optical stylet
	McGrath "AIRCRAFT"	Res-Q-Scope II			
	GlideScope				
Storz V-Mac	Storz D-Blade				
	King Vision				
	Venner A.P. Advance				
	MedAn				

Table 1. Summary of different types of VL devices.

with no antifogging mechanism. It has the longest intubation time among other video techniques and higher learning curve but is very useful in restricted mouth opening using retromolar space. The Shikani optical stylet is a malleable, stainless steel, J-shaped endoscope with illumination fibers and a fiberoptic bundle that can be used with a separate camera and monitor system, or on its own with an optical eyepiece. **Figure 1** shows Bonfils retromolar videolaryngoscope.

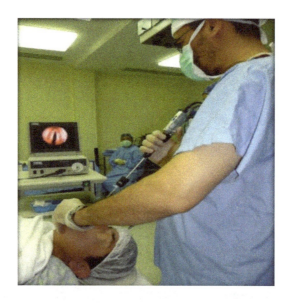

Figure 1. Bonfils retromolar videolaryngoscope (Storz-Company).

3.3.2. Channeled videolaryngoscopy

The representatives of the family are Pentax and AirTraq. All channeled devices have been designed mainly for oral intubation; however, the recent version of AirTraq has been studied and used in nasal intubation. The AirTraq is a single-use optical device with optional video camera attachment. It is available in different sizes and could be used for nasal intubation and double lumen tube insertion; however, it is single use and it requires 30–40 s to reduce fogging. Pentax is similar to AirTraq, with the advantage of the only plastic guide blades which are disposable. The tip is angled by 135° and it cannot be used with an endotracheal tube (ETT) less than 6.5, making it impractical for pediatric population. Both Pentax and AirTraq have been proved to reduce the cervical spine mobility in patients with unstable cervical spine or reduced spinal mobility. Res-Q-Scope is a similar device, but the clinical studies are so limited.

3.3.3. Rigid blades

Rigid blades are classified into standard blade or angled blade. In general, the standard blades use the various modifications of typical Macintosh blades as C-Mac (**Figure 2**). However, the angled blades offer more angulations near the distal tip to widen the view angle. In some equipment, as in Coopdech D-scope, sizes of 0,1 and Miller's blades are available, etc. C-scope sizes (sizes 0 and 1) Miller blades are available, but in most of the others Macintosh blades sizes 2, 3, and 4 are the standard.

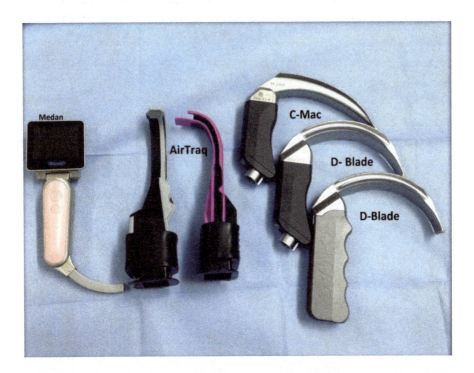

Figure 2. Videolaryngoscopes.

It was shown that the design familiarity with standard Macintosh blades, side screen, and enhanced view has reduced the learning curve for the inexperienced providers.

The main difference among rigid blades is the blade angulation and the position of the side view screen. In Coopdech VLP100, it has a build-in screen on top of the device with the view angle of 39-52°, with the option of sizes 2, 3, and 4 Macintosh or size 0, 1 Miller blade. The McGrath "AIRCRAFT" is similar to Coopdech VLP100 in having a build-in side screen over the handle, but different in having adjustable variable length blades that snaps in place once the length is adjusted. The GlideScope (**Figure 3**) has an angulation of 60°, with antifogging camera, plastic disposable blades, and separate view screen. GlideScope appeared to be the most intuitive, easy to learn with the steepest learning curve [11] but a little bit bulky in relation to C-Mac blade; that is why most of clinicians prefer C-Mac over GlideScope. Venner A.P. Advance and MedAn videolaryngoscopes are also available in the market from these VL types but the clinical studies are so limited.

In general, not one device has shown to have a 100% success rate and none has shown to be superior to another. All studies concluded that VL offers better laryngoscopic view if not the same as direct laryngoscopy. Most of the studies have concluded that the intubation time is more with videolaryngoscopy than with the direct laryngoscopy. Relative devices were faster than others by few seconds, DCI Storz Videolaryngoscope is relatively faster by 10 s than GlideScope (34 s) and McGarth (38 s); other study showed that the time for intubation for GlideScope was 33 s, CMAC was 17 s, and McGarth was 41 s [12]. Intubation with the GlideScope has been found to be 99% successful after initial failure of direct laryngoscopy, helping to reduce the incidence of failed intubation. It should be noted that the relative learning curves could affect the performance of GlideScope in some studies, as in

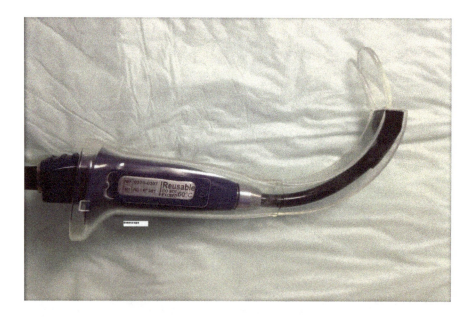

Figure 3. GlideScope (Verathon Inc., US).

the study of Platts-Mills in emergency department, which showed no difference in intubation failure between GlideScope and Macintosh, and intubation time in GlideScope was longer (12 s) [13] (**Figure 3**).

The main advantage for the videolaryngoscopy is minimal cervical spine mobility during intubation as the pharyngeal and laryngeal axis should not align together, offering least mobility for cervical instability. Moreover, it is helpful in case of limited accessibility, for example, magnetic resonance imaging (MRI) scanning, beach chair position, or prone position. It also allows sharing the airway view with beyond the operator for teaching or assistance purposes (**Figure 2**).

The devices of VL have been evaluated and adopted for practice outside the operative room.

3.4. Disadvantages of VL

The most common disadvantages of VL could be variable learning curve that depends on the level of training and experience, difficult passage of tube despite satisfactory laryngeal view, and loss of the depth perception. The fogging and secretion that could obstruct the camera are among other technical issues. Other disadvantage is the cost that could range from 5000 to 10,000$, which could be a burden in some part of the world; however, the cost could be justifiable in the industrialized part of the world if it could prevent such fatal airway events with its subsequent million dollar lawsuits. One study for VL adoption in Massachusetts emergency departments in 2012 has showed that adoption rate for VL was 43%, a relatively fast rate. The 69% of non-adopters have attributed that to the cost of the device [14].

4. Flexible fiberoptic intubation in ICU

4.1. Introduction

It is an airway device used for indirect visualization of the airway either for airway management or for other diagnostic and therapeutic purposes. Traditionally, all old scopes have used the fiberoptic fiber technology; however, the newer scopes, out of reliability issues, do not use the fiberoptic technology anymore and that's why the nomenclature changed to flexible intubation scope.

4.2. Types

Flexible intubation scope is a flexible cord that has fiberoptic fibers (old scopes) or optical fibers with a small camera on the tip of the scope using complementary metal oxide semiconductor (CMOS) technology and the so-called flexible intubation video endoscope (FIVE) from Storz Company. The proximal handle has a working channel port for oxygen and suction, lever to flex or extend the tip and light source. The diameter of adult scope is of 3.8 and 4.2 mm which can hold ETT of 6.5 mm or more. The diameter of children scope is of 2.2 and 3.1 mm which can hold 3 and 4 mm EET, respectively. Both adult and pediatric scopes have working channel of 1.2 mm. Most of flexible intubation scopes are reusable; however, recently a single-use flexible intubation scope started to be in the market from Ambu Company.

4.3. Indications

The main indication of flexible scope intubation (FSI) in anesthesia care and ICU settings is to secure the placement of endotracheal tube when there is anticipated airway difficulty and confirmation of tube position after intubation if necessary. It can be used as well in the management of abnormal airway anatomy, obstructive upper airway lesion, and unstable cervical spine to limit the cervical mobility, and the evaluation of airway obstruction is another anesthetic indication as a preoperative assessment (preoperative naso-endoscopy in pre-assessment anesthesia clinic) or directly prior to intubation for the patients with known anatomical abnormalities in the upper airway. The choice of the route has its indications as well, as nasal route is used in a case of limited mouth opening or a strong gag reflex, or if the surgery needs nasal intubation. Other indications other than primary anesthetic care involve diagnostic and therapeutic purposes, see **Table 2**.

4.4. Contraindications

There are no absolute contraindications for the FSI, but in the following situations difficult to impossible scenarios could be encountered. Large airway bleeding and secretions could make the view impossible. The limited clinical experience of the operator, the necessities for rapid airway control, the need to insert the tube under vision to minimize further trauma to the upper airway, and uncooperative patient are other contraindications. However, it is not absolute, as uncooperative patient can be intubated as sleep FSI and the visualization for ETT

Diagnostic indications	Therapeutic indications
• Evaluation of pneumonia, atelectasis, infiltrate of unclear etiology.	• Mucus impaction.
• Evaluation of hemoptysis.	• Foreign body removal.
• Evaluation of toxic burn inhalation.	• Laser coagulation for lesions.
• Evaluation of chest trauma.	• Photodynamic therapy.
• Evaluation of chronic cough.	• Electrocoagulation.
• Placement of artificial airways.	• Cryotherapy.
• Evaluate complications of tracheostomy.	• Dilation by balloon.
• Evaluation of precancerous lesions.	• Brachytherapy.
• Evaluation of tracheoesophageal fistula.	• Tracheobronchial stents.
• Evaluation of bronchopleural fistula.	• Bronchopleural fistula.
• Confocal microbronchoscopy.	• Needle aspiration of mediastinal cysts.

Table 2. Indications of flexible scope intubation (FSI).

insertion could be achieved by adjuvant airway as in fiberoptic-assisted videoscopic intubation (FAVI), a technique, when other indirect visualization technique, as C-Mac VL (**Figure 2**), is used to facilitate the insertion of ETT under vision. Nasal route is contraindicated in case of severe craniofacial deformity and skull base fracture.

4.5. Preparation for flexible scope intubation (FSI)

The preparation step for FSI is the most important step for a successful procedure. It involves patient selection and preparation, airway anesthesia and equipment preparation. The patient selection will determine whether the FSI will be through the oral or nasal route and whether it will be awake or sleep FSI. Generally, the awake has better visualization than the deep, due to loss of muscle tone and pharyngeal collapse after induction of anesthesia.

4.5.1. Patient preparation

It starts by good communication with the patient and proper assessment of the underlying condition. Anti-sialagogues should be applied for all patients whether it is oral or nasal, as secretions do not only affect the view but also limit the action of the local anesthetics. Commonly, it is recommended to use intravenous 0.2 mg glycopyrrolate, 15 min before the procedure. For patients with high risk for aspiration, risk and benefit should be analyzed as airway anesthesia and long intubation time could compromise the airway reflexes and increase aspiration risk. Certain measures have been recommended to minimize that risk: as intubation in head-up position, administration of 0.3 M sodium citrate 30 ml and Metoclopramide 10 mg or Ranitidine 50 mg within 1 h before the start of the procedure. Patient positioning depends on the technique and patient and operator's preference as well. Positions could be sitting (beach-chair), lateral decubitus for awake FSI or supine positions for sleep FSI and prone position as a rescue technique.

Airway anesthesia is a critical step in the procedure. It can be done by applying the local anesthetic solutions, gel, or ointment by atomizer, nebulizer, or "spray as you go technique." Airway anesthesia equipment includes atomizing devices, nebulizers, syringes and needles, and cotton swabs.

Combined techniques are always recommended to optimize the outcome. Combination of 4% lidocaine nebulization, atomization spray to tongue, and oropharynx followed by "spray as you go" through the working channel of the scope using epidural catheter are commonly applied together.

Cautions should be taken not to exceed with the lidocaine dosage above 6 mg/kg to avoid systemic toxicity. Trans-tracheal local anesthetic infiltration and nerve blocks could be used with a skilled operator but it is not commonly done. Glossopharyngeal nerve block, superior laryngeal nerve block, sphenopalatine nerve block, and anterior ethmoidal nerve block are among the nerves that could be blocked; however, the discussion of each nerve technique will be beyond the scope of this chapter. For nasal anesthesia, vasoconstrictors as 1% phenylephrine or 0.05% oxymetazoline are added to the local anesthetics to minimize nasal bleeding.

Airway equipment includes flexible intubating scope, face mask, specialized oral airway, and endotracheal tube, antifogging agent, lubricating agent, nasopharyngeal airway, oral or nasal mucosal atomization device (MAD) and video monitor. All equipment should be checked for functionality before any operation.

4.6. Technique

Oral intubation is the most common route. Stepwise approach should be followed: as ETT is loaded first to the scope, then oropharyngeal suction before insertion of scope, then applying of bite blocker or fiberoptic plastic airway (e.g., Ovassapian, Williams, or Berman). FSI should always be in the midline till satisfactory view is achieved. The working channel offers a source for suction, oxygen insufflation, or channel for epidural catheter during the procedure.

Nasal intubation has its advantage in avoiding the gag reflex; however, the chance of epistaxis is high. Topical nasal decongestant such as 0.05% oxymetazoline and 1% phenylephrine should be used to decrease the nasal mucosal irritation and bleeding.

Awake intubation necessitates patient cooperation, adequate airway anesthesia; however, sedation may be required. The patient is asked to swallow or breathe deeply and smoothly. Sedation could be titrated on individual basis, based on the underlying comorbidities. Commonly used sedation is Remifentanil infusion starting with 0.05 μg/kg/min or Remifentanil target-controlled infusion (TCI) mode with or without 1–2 mg Midazolam or Dexmedetomidine 0.3 μg/kg/h with or without Midazolam 1–2 mg or incremental doses of Midazolam 1 mg alone. Propofol TCI is another alternative to Midazolam as a sedative agent.

Sleep intubation could be done after induction of anesthesia in certain circumstances.

4.7. Strategies for success

It is important to keep in mind that FSI is a complex clinical procedure with requirements of special skills, which make even good preparation not enough to guarantee the success. Practicing certain adjuvant measures as strategies for enhancing the laryngoscopic view and facilitated ETT insertion could decrease the failure rate. Enhancing the view could be achieved by keeping airway patent by one or more of the following: jaw thrust, pulling tongue out by a gauze, fiberoptic oral airway placement, external laryngeal manipulation, insertion of laryngoscopic blade with lifting the epiglottis away from the pharyngeal wall (VAFI technique), and clearing the lens fogging by gentle touch of mucus membrane. Facilitated ETT insertion aims to minimize a possible trauma from the blind insertion of the tube after the FIS has reached the carina. The facilitation could be done by a 90° anticlockwise rotation of the tube to avoid getting caught at right arytenoid, warming the tube, flexible tube and combination of direct and indirect laryngoscopic technique or using video-assisted fiberoptic intubation (VAFI) technique.

4.8. Advantages

Flexible intubation scope is unique airway visualization equipment that offers great clinical help, not only in the management of difficult airway scenarios but also in the diagnosis and treatment as well. More details are described under bronchoscopy section.

4.9. Disadvantages

FSI is a complex procedure with no straightforward steps. To master the technique, it requires a lot of practice with high learning curve. Extra equipments are always necessary; moreover, it requires time for preparation and cannot help in emergency situation. Nasal epistaxis, minor airway trauma as erythema, and vocal cord injury could occur.

5. Bronchoscopy in ICU

5.1. Introduction

Flexible fiberoptic bronchoscopy is frequently used for diagnosis and therapy, performed in ventilated patients via an endo-tracheal tube or tracheostomy tube in ICU and other critical areas. Indication may be diagnostic or therapeutic (**Table 2**). *The most common indications* include clearance of retained secretion, mucous plug, lung collapse, endobronchial brush, removal of blood clot, diagnosis of ventilator-associated pneumonia by broncho-alveolar lavage (BAL), trans-bronchial biopsy, detection of airway lesions (e.g., neoplastic), endobronchial ultrasound (US), and visualization of instruments during percutaneous tracheostomy. Contraindications are relative so each patient should be carefully assessed for risk benefits. *Contraindications* include uncooperative patient, unstable patient as severe hypoxemia, hypercarbia, unstable asthma, recent myocardial infarction, or any situation of possible serious hemorrhage after biopsy as uremia, tracheal obstruction or stenosis and pulmonary hypertension.

5.2. Management of the airway for bronchoscopy

Separate operator should manage airway and ventilation. The bronchoscopist should be prepared to interrupt the procedure immediately if there is destabilization. Patients are pre-oxygenated, anesthetized, paralyzed, and ventilated on 100% O_2. Positive end expiratory pressure (PEEP) should be maintained. Impairment of gas exchange is common due to tube obstruction and when suction is applied through the scope.

Endotracheal tubes smaller than 8-mm internal diameter may be significantly occluded by flexible fiberoptic bronchoscopy and this could impair ventilation and oxygenation. A lubricated swivel (or elbow) connector with a fitted rubber cap prevents loss of ventilation. If pressure-controlled ventilation is used, peak pressure setting should be increased to compensate for the loss of tidal volume. Suction periods should be limited to 5 s or less. Thick secretions often require instillation of saline (10–20 ml) down the injection port to dissolve them. During broncho-alveolar lavage (BAL), a sputum trap should be used between bronchoscope and wall suction.

5.3. Special situation with flexible fiberoptic bronchoscopy

- *Bleeding dyscrasias:* Coagulation studies, platelet counts, and hemoglobin concentration are necessary before the procedure especially when there are clinical risk factors for abnormal coagulation. Bronchoscopy with lavage can be performed with platelet counts of >20,000 per/µl.

- *Pneumothorax:* A chest radiograph should be obtained if a patient is symptomatic or if there is a clinical suspicion of possible pneumothorax after trans-bronchial biopsy. Patients should be advised of the potential for delayed complications following trans-bronchial biopsy.

- *Fever and infection:* Antibiotic prophylaxis is not warranted before bronchoscopy for the prevention of endocarditis, fever, or pneumonia.

- *Ischemic heart disease:* flexible fiberoptic bronchoscopy should ideally be delayed for 4 weeks after MI.

6. Percutaneous tracheostomy

6.1. Introduction

Mechanical ventilation can be delivered to the patient who requires ventilatory support either initially through endotracheal tube (ETT) for short-term period or through tracheostomy tube, in cases where the respiratory support will be prolonged due to underlying medical reasons [15].

Tracheostomy versus intubation: The relative advantages and disadvantages of tracheostomy and endotracheal intubation are outlined in **Table 3** [16–20].

Tracheostomy techniques: Bedside percutaneous tracheostomy is an alternative to operative (open) tracheostomy, as it could be done either at the bedside or in the operating room. Successful performance of the bedside percutaneous procedure is related to the expertise of the operator and supportive personnel. Surgeons or well-trained critical care clinicians could do with fewer complications. Choosing between open or percutaneous tracheostomy depends upon the availability of each procedure and institutional expertise.

	Intubation	Tracheostomy
Advantage	• Highly skilled personnel are required.	• Ability to speech, swallowing.
	• Stoma complication is less.	• Ability to mobile and discharged outside ICU.
	• Procedural complication is less.	• Easy suction.
		• Better patient satisfaction and comfort.
Disadvantage	• Possible mouth, nasal or laryngeal injury.	• Cuff pressure complication.
	• Cuff pressure complication.	• Stoma and fistula complications.
	• Requirement of tube exchange or possible ICU care.	• Possible laryngeal injury, pulmonary and mediastinum complication.
		• Mortality complication due de-cannulation in improper time.

Table 3. Advantage and disadvantage tracheostomy versus intubation.

Percutaneous versus operative: Percutaneous tracheostomy offers numerous advantages compared to operative tracheostomy: it requires less time to perform, it is less expensive, and it is typically performed sooner (because an operating room doesn't have to be scheduled). In addition, overall complications may be less frequent with percutaneous tracheostomy than surgical tracheostomy, even though percutaneous tracheostomy has an increased risk of anterior tracheal injury and posterior tracheal wall perforation.

Data describing outcomes comparing both techniques are conflicting, which may reflect the different techniques used to perform percutaneous tracheostomy (e.g., ultrasound-guided, bronchoscopy-guided, dilatational, other).

6.2. Complication

Infection: In two meta-analyses of randomized controlled trials, percutaneous dilatational tracheostomy reduced wound infections (e.g., odds ratio: 0.28, 95% CI: 0.16–0.49) compared to both surgical tracheostomy performed in the ICU and surgical tracheostomy performed in the operating room. A separate meta-analysis of 29 randomized and non-randomized studies reported a similar reduction in the rate of wound infection with percutaneous tracheostomy [21].

Bleeding and mortality: When compared to surgical tracheostomy performed in the operating room, only percutaneous dilatational tracheostomy has also been associated with reduced bleeding (odds ratio: 0.29, 95% CI: 0.12–0.75) and mortality (odds ratio: 0.71, 95% CI: 0.50–1.0). A similar reduction in overall mortality was reported in another 10-year review of 616 trauma patients that compared those who underwent percutaneous tracheostomy with those who underwent open tracheostomy (10 vs. 15%) [17].

By contrast, another meta-analysis of 20 trials reported no difference in mortality or major bleeding [18]. In a separate meta-analysis, perioperative complications (including death, serious cardiorespiratory events, and minor complications) were rare, but more common with percutaneous tracheostomy than with surgical tracheostomy. In another meta-analysis of 29 studies, no significant difference in bleeding or tracheal stenosis was reported [20].

Scarring: While one meta-analysis reported no difference in the rate of tracheal stenosis or scarring, another reported significant reduction on the rate of scarring.

Taken together, the data suggest that percutaneous dilatational tracheostomy offers numerous advantages compared to surgical tracheostomy. However, the benefit of percutaneous tracheostomy may be substantially less dependent upon the technique employed.

6.3. Contraindications

Relative contraindications to percutaneous tracheostomy include age under 15 years of age; uncorrectable bleeding diathesis; gross distortion of the neck from hematoma, tumor, thyroid gland enlargement, or scarring from previous neck surgery; documented or clinically suspected tracheomalacia; evidence of infection in the soft tissues of the neck; obese and/or short neck which obscures landmarks; and inability to extend the neck because of cervical fusion, rheumatoid arthritis, or other causes of cervical spine instability.

It should be reiterated that these contraindications are relative. Percutaneous dilatational tracheostomy has been performed successfully by skilled operators in patients who were very old, were morbidly obese, had a history of previous tracheostomy, or had thrombocytopenia (the patients received pre-procedure platelet transfusions). It has also been performed successfully in patients receiving high-frequency oscillation ventilation or positive end expiratory pressure (PEEP) at a level of >10 cm H_2O.

A study that evaluated the rates of bleeding complications during percutaneous tracheostomy showed that bleeding complications could be predicted by a platelet count less than 50,000/µl, an activated partial thromboplastin time longer than 50 s, or the presence of two or more coagulation disorders. Administration of prophylactic subcutaneous heparin did not increase the risk of bleeding [18].

For patients undergoing a bronchoscopic-guided percutaneous tracheostomy, a bedside checklist, similar to that performed for open tracheostomy performed in the operating room, may be associated with reduced procedural complications.

6.4. Complications

Acute: The most common acute (e.g., first few days) complications include obstruction and pneumothorax as well as postoperative hemorrhage and infection.

Obstruction: Percutaneous tracheostomy tubes can become partially obstructed by the posterior membranous trachea following initial placement, although symptomatic obstruction is uncommon. This complication appears to be related to the experience of the clinician performing the procedure. However, the swelling of the posterior tracheal wall could cause symptomatic compression of the tube up to 1 week after placement.

Subcutaneous emphysema and pneumothorax: The incidence of subcutaneous emphysema and pneumothorax is 1.4 and 0.8%, respectively [19]. Cadaver models revealed that imperfect positioning of fenestrated cannula and posterior wall perforation are possible mechanisms for these complications [19].

Chronic complications of tracheostomy (i.e., weeks and months) that are specific to tracheostomy include the following:

- *Tracheal stenosis:* Granulation tissue is the main reason for tracheal obstruction in patients under long mechanical ventilation by tracheostomy, which differs from the stenosis that develops in endotracheal tube that will be appearing earlier and be web-like. Stenosis of the trachea is not only below the tracheostomy tube, but it may occur above the tracheal stoma but below the glottis. That could contribute to high-peak airway pressures and difficulty in weaning. Treatment includes the placement of a longer tracheostomy tube, surgical intervention, or the placement of a tracheal stent [20].

- *Tracheoarterial fistula:* Massive hemorrhage due to a tracheoarterial fistula is the most devastating complication. Tracheoarterial fistula (most often a tracheoinnominate artery fistula) was more common in the past from low-positioned tracheostomy tubes and is now rarely encountered with several studies reporting an incidence of <1% in both short-term and long-term tracheostomies [21]. The development of a tracheoarterial fistula is a life-threatening complication with a reported survival of 14%. Tracheoarterial fistulas are due to erosion from the tube tip or cuff into the anterior wall of the trachea resulting in a fistulous communication with the innominate artery as it passes anteriorly across the trachea. Patients may develop a "sentinel" bleeding followed by massive hemoptysis. Diagnosis is dependent upon a high index of suspicion, and when suspected, immediate action should be undertaken to stop the bleeding since diagnostic modalities such as angiography or bronchoscopy may lead to delay and death.

The following temporizing maneuvers may be performed while waiting for definitive therapy, which is surgical repair [22].

- In an attempt to compress the innominate artery, the tracheostomy or endotracheal tube cuff may be overinflated.

- If the above fails, an ETT may be placed orally, the tracheostomy removed, and the cuff inflated distal to the tracheostomy site.

- If that fails, a finger can be placed through the tracheostomy stoma and positioned distally into the trachea ("The little Dutch boy maneuver"); the finger is then pulled anteriorly to compress the artery against the sternum (pressure should be sufficient to lift the torso anteriorly). Pressure should be maintained during transport to the operating room. Ventilation and oxygenation need to be preserved with a bag-valve mask or intubation with an ETT orally.

Reduced phonation: Following tracheostomy, many patients experience a reduction in or loss of phonation, the duration of which may be prolonged or indefinite, and the effect of which can be devastating to some patients. Traditionally, speech valves are used in tracheostomized patients (with the cuff deflated) who successfully wean from mechanical ventilation and are able to self-ventilate. Preliminary data suggest that early phonation is feasible and may be beneficial when instituted during mechanical ventilation in tracheostomized patients. As an example, one randomized trial of 30 ventilated tracheostomized patients reported that early intervention with cuff deflation plus an in-line speaking valve during mechanical ventilation shortened the time to phonation by 11 days, when compared with late intervention using the standard approach. Further research is needed before in-line speaking valves can become routine for this population [22].

Others: Tracheoesophageal fistula is more commonly encountered with prolonged endotracheal intubation and is discussed separately.

Although not studied in a randomized trial, the complication rate associated with tracheostomy may be increased in obese patients with a body mass index of ≥35 [22].

Changing a tracheostomy tube: There are no universally accepted indications for changing a tracheostomy tube. Therefore, the following indications are based on clinical experience rather than on empirical evidence:

Routine changes: Tracheostomy tubes are routinely changed from 7 to 14 days after initial insertion and then every 60 to 90 days. Observational data suggest that changing the tracheostomy tube before 7 days may be associated with earlier use of a speaking valve and earlier ability to tolerate oral intake. A consensus statement recommends changing the tracheostomy tube at 3–7 days if inserted operatively but 10–14 days if placed via the percutaneous dilatational method.

Patient discomfort: Patient discomfort may respond to a reduction in the size of the tracheostomy tube.

Malposition: Tracheostomy tube malposition may respond to a change in the length or size of the tracheostomy tube.

Patient-ventilator asynchrony: Patient-ventilator asynchrony that is related to the tracheostomy tube may respond to changing the tube.

Cuff leak: A cuff leak may be due to malposition of the tracheostomy tube (particularly in the setting of tracheomalacia) and may respond to changing the tube.

Fracture: Fracture of the tracheostomy tube or flange is an indication for a new tracheostomy tube.

Type change: Changing a tracheostomy tube from one type to another may be indicated by the clinical circumstances; as an example, changing from a balloon cuff to either a foam cuff or a cuff-less tracheostomy tube.

Bronchoscopy: Flexible bronchoscopy generally requires a tracheostomy tube with an inner diameter of at least 7.5 mm; thus, the tracheostomy tube may need to be changed to one with a larger inner diameter to facilitate bronchoscopy.

Decannulation: Appropriate candidates for tracheal decannulation after weaning from mechanical ventilation include patients who fulfill all the following criteria:

No upper airway obstruction, ability to clear secretions that are neither too copious nor too thick, and presence of an effective cough. In patients with neuromuscular disease, a peak cough flow greater than 160 ml/min generally predicts successful decannulation. The value of this measurement in patients without neuromuscular disease is unknown.

Failed decannulation has been associated with age, greater severity of illness, the presence of renal failure, and a shorter duration of spontaneous breathing prior to decannulation or the insertion of a tracheostomy plug.

7. Extubation in ICU

7.1. Introduction

The removal of endotracheal tube (ETT) termed as extubation is the last step of ventilatory weaning. Extubation step necessitates consideration of patient condition, experience with extubation techniques, and post-extubation management.

Before extubation: Successful weaning from mechanical support is not the only prerequisite for safe extubation. Extubation is carried on patent airway with adequate airway reflex after independence from ventilatory support.

Airway protection: Airway protection requires a conscious patient with a strong cough reflex and minimal secretions.

Typical criteria for successful weaning: Fully awake and cooperative, good muscle tone and function, intact bulbar function, stable hemodynamic, no dysrhythmias, Hb greater than 8.0 gm%, minimal inotropic requirements, optimal fluid balance, respiratory $FiO_2 < 0.4$, PEEP < 10 cm H_2O, no significant respiratory acidosis (PH > 7.3 or $PaCO_2$ <6.5 kPa), good cough, normal metabolic pH, normal electrolyte balance, non-distended abdomen, adequate nutritional status, normal CO_2 production, and normal oxygen demands [23].

Some patients will be extubated without difficulty and others will rapidly deteriorate as a result of inadequate respiratory effort or clearance of secretions. Those patients will require re-intubation, ventilation, and another period of optimization and consideration for tracheostomy. Some patients will benefit from weaning straight onto mask CPAP or NIV [23].

Difficult extubation: Extubation of a patient with a known difficult airway requires careful planning in anticipation for potential re-intubation. If there are doubts about airway patency prior to extubation, then direct laryngoscopy, fiberoptic bronchoscopy, and assessment of leak upon cuff deflation are useful checks. Patients who are considered likely to be difficult to re-intubate can be extubated with an airway exchange catheter in situ, to allow rapid re-intubation. Intravenous dexamethasone, nebulized adrenaline, and Heliox have been used with variable success in such circumstances.

Risk factors for extubation failure are peak expiratory flow rate (PEFR) of ≤ 60 L/min, sputum volume production of > 2.5 ml/h, and compromised neurological status. Combination of three risk factors reliably predicts extubation failure by 100% compared to 3% if no risk factor mentioned above is present [24].

Post-extubation management: Post-extubation care includes suctioning, bronchodilator therapy, diuresis, or noninvasive ventilation (NIV). Those measures could aid to prevent re-intubation by improving the oxygenation and airway clearance.

Oxygen (including high-flow nasal cannula (HFNC)): Every patient should be oxygenated post-extubation. We prefer using devices that provide adequate oxygenation and comfort for the patient. For most patients, this goal is achieved with low-flow devices (nasal prongs, simple, or venturi face masks). When higher flows of oxygen are required, high-flow nasal cannula (HFNC) may offer improved oxygenation, provide a small amount of positive end expiratory pressure (PEEP), and is better tolerated when compared with oxygen delivered through low- or high-flow face masks.

The efficacy of HFNC in the post-extubation setting was best illustrated in a trial of 527 patients who were mechanically ventilated for an average of only 1–2 days and considered to be at low risk for re-intubation following extubation. Compared to conventional low-flow oxygen therapy, HFNC reduced the rate of re-intubation at 72 h (5 vs. 12%) as well as the rate of respiratory failure (14 vs. 8%). However, methodologic flaws such as imperfect blinding and the high proportion of postsurgical and neurologic patients, where HFNC may have improved secretion clearance, may have biased results in favor of HFNC. Although encouraging, this trial does not support the routine use of HFNC following extubation [25].

In addition, while further studies are required to clarify who benefits the most from HFNC after extubation, its use in those who are severely hypoxemic is appropriate (e.g., partial arterial pressure of oxygen/fraction of inspired oxygen ratio <300). Further details regarding HNFC in other medical and postoperative populations and efficacy compared with NIV in post-extubation patients are discussed separately.

8. High-flow nasal cannula (HFNC)

8.1. Introduction

Different names and descriptions of this therapy:

HFNC: **H**igh-**F**low **N**asal **C**annula.

THRIVE: **T**rans**n**asal **H**umidified **R**apid **I**nsufflation **V**entilatory **E**xchange.

POINT: **P**erioperative **O**xygenation **I**nsufflatory **N**asal **T**herapy (**Figure 4**).

Or transnasal insufflation or nasal high-flow or nasal high-flow ventilation or high-flow therapy or high-flow nasal cannula oxygen therapy.

HFNC oxygen delivery system involves a mixture of oxygen/air, an active humidified, heated circuit, and nasal cannula. The active heater and humidifier are able to deliver heated and humidified high flow reaching 60 L/min than has many physiological advantages. High flow is able to reduce dead space by maintaining PEEP inside the airway and supplying constant fraction of oxygen. In spite of limited evidence in literature in ICU, it has gained popularity among physicians in various critical conditions. The existing evidence in neonates proves that HFNC decreases the work of breathing by reducing the respiratory rate and sufficiently supports the patient ventilation, reducing the escalation of ventilator support [26].

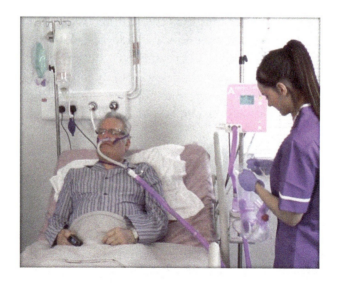

Figure 4. High-flow nasal cannula (HFNC) (Aqua VENT FD 140® from Armstrong Medical Company, Northern Ireland).

As the evidence is still evolving, still the indications and contraindications should be considered for each case individually.

8.2. Indications

- Hypercapnic respiratory failure.
- Hypoxemic respiratory failure.
- Post-extubation.
- Pre-intubation oxygenation.
- Sleep apnea.
- Acute heart failure.

8.3. Contraindication

- Bilateral nasal blockade as postnasal operations.
- Nasal bleeding.
- Nasal tumors.
- Nasal infection.
- It is also unlikely that HFNC can readily rescue those patients who have total airway obstruction and its use in the presence of a known or suspected cranial base fracture is also not advised.

8.4. Advantages

- Better tolerated in some patients than face masks.
- Fixed performance, permitting accurate delivery of up to 100% oxygen in most clinical situations.
- Gas is warmed and humidified.
- Low-level positive airways pressure is possible.
- An additional benefit is that nasal high-flow devices have been shown to produce positive airway pressures of over 5 cm H_2O, thus permitting their use in place of low-level CPAP [26].
- It is an open system and we do not have to care about the tight contact of interfaces, and HFNC can be applicable to patients with claustrophobia.

8.5. Disadvantages

- Results of large-scale clinical trials are still awaited.

- More expensive than standard oxygen delivery devices.
- Not yet available in all hospitals, and rarely outside of critical care.

9. Usage of supraglottic airway devices (SGAD) in ICU

9.1. Introduction

Airway management in the critical care is challenging and differs from the operating theatre. The supra-glottic airway devices (SGADs), especially the laryngeal mask airway (LMA), provide a fast and lifesaving way in the critical events.

9.2. Advantages

- Can solve "Cannot Intubate, Cannot Ventilate" (CICV) scenario.
- Passing a Bougie through it, then intubation over a Bougie or using an Aintree Intubating Catheter (Cook Critical Care, Bloomington, IN, USA).
- Bronchoscopy through LMA.
- Used as an airway while performing a tracheostomy.
- Ventilation during cardiac arrest instead of an ETT, if no skilled staffs are available.
- Minimal skills requirements to use an LMA.
- No muscle relaxant is required.
- No contact with vocal cords, less irritating than ETT.

9.3. Disadvantages

- No guarantee for a good airway, as the tip may fold on itself blocking the airway.
- No good seal with no protection from aspiration.
- Intubating through the LMA could be problematic. As it has shown that the LMA opening sits perfectly above the cords only in 45–60% of the time [27]. This means almost half of the time the LMA is directing the ETT away from the cords. The situation is worse in difficult airway as the provider was perfectly capable of shoving the tube the wrong way without any help.

9.4. Evidence for and against the use of LMAs in critical care

- Experts have recommended the use of LMA in a "Cannot Intubate, Cannot Ventilate" (CICV) scenario while waiting for a better airway. It has shown that LMAs have saved lives in such situations [28].

- The dilemma of LMAs not offering a good seal has no effect on clinical outcomes. Risk of aspiration has never been demonstrated, even with the old generations of LMA [29].

- No difference between the LMA and routine bag-mask and ETT anesthesia [29]

- Using the LMA as an airway while performing a tracheostomy has no sufficient evidence in the literature. There is no difference in the rate of complications, but the tracheostomies involving LMAs seemed to be quicker, may be due to less time to adjust the ETT cuff above the cords [30].

10. Endotracheal tube exchanger in ICU

10.1. Indications

- Mostly due to a cuff leak.

- The need for a different endotracheal tube (ETT) size as when smaller one is needed in patients with vocal cord edema or larger ETT for flexible bronchoscopy procedure.

- Change of special types of ETT like reinforced or double lumen to ordinary ETT.

10.2. Complications

However, exchanging the ETT may be life-threatening and lead to

- Esophageal intubation.

- Loss of the airway.

- Severe hypoxia.

- Cardiac arrest.

The risk may be more in those with a difficult airway or those with poor cardiopulmonary reserve.

10.3. Techniques

The ideal way for ETT exchange has not yet been studied. Experienced team with advanced airway skills should be consulted priorv to ETT replacement.

The ETT placement can be done under direct laryngoscopy or indirect laryngoscopy with or without a Bougie guide. The initial airway assessment by direct laryngoscopy will determine which tool should be used. When a good laryngeal view is obtained by direct laryngoscopy, ETT can be introduced safely; however, in difficult laryngeal view, video laryngoscopy should be sought. Intubation medications are recommended to be used as well in tube exchange. Video laryngoscopy has been shown, compared with historical controls, to reduce the number of attempts at ETT exchange, with fewer complications including hypoxemia, esophageal intubation, bradycardia, and need for rescue airway device intervention [31].

11. Virtual endoscopy and 3D reconstruction of airway

Virtual endoscopy (VE) (**Figure 5**) is a noninvasive technology by which two-dimensional (2D) or three-dimensional (3D) images are reconstructed by computer software from high-resolution computed tomography (CT) scan (**Figure 6**). Virtual bronchoscopy was initially reported in 1993, but it was modified in 1996 to be used in virtual laryngoscopy. The virtual images reconstructed by software have comparable quality of fiberoptic views with sensitivity of 100% to detect upper airway lesions [32, 33]. The novel application of virtual laryngoscopy is eminent in the assessment and staging of upper airway lesion, comprehensive preoperative airway assessment, and planning of complex reconstructive upper airway surgeries. The "fly-through" reconstructions provided accurate and comparable images to fiberoptic bronchoscopy, which provided valuable information for the evaluation of the airway passages in a step forward prior to going to the difficult airway management (**Figure 5**). The utilization of the 3D imaging package is now commercially available within the workstation delivered by the different vendors worldwide, to obtain 3D models of the airway. This approach will be the added value and advantage that most anesthetists and intensive care physician would be able to use this technology to construct VE images of the airway from existing CT images and find them easy to interpret (**Figure 7**).

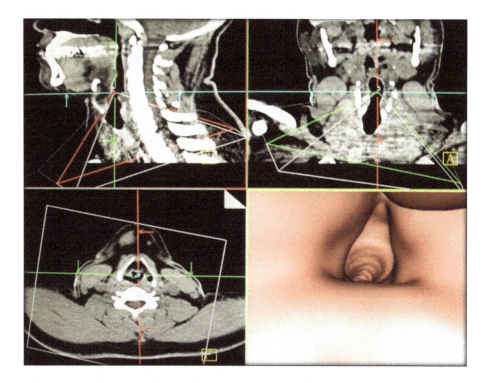

Figure 5. Virtual endoscopic evaluation of the air way. The vocal cords are well demonstrated. The accompanied reference images in axial, coronal, and sagittal planes with the virtual endoscope are noted, and its apex represents the eyepiece while the base represents the virtual lens.

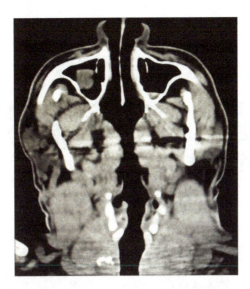

Figure 6. Curved MPR multi-planar reconstruction of the airway showing the entire airway in single plane from the nares down to the trachea allowing accurate measurement and orientation of the airway caliber at the different levels.

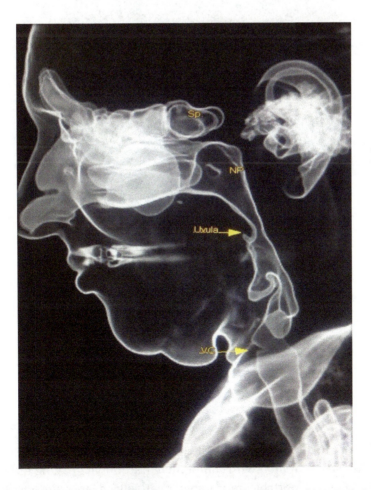

Figure 7. Lateral projections of the SSD-shaded surface display using volume-rendering techniques for the airway. SP: sphenoid sinus; NS: nasopharynx; VC: vocal cord.

This state-of-the-art technology has a promising future value in airway management for both anesthesiologists and intensivists as they will be able to easily interpret the airway images by noninvasive way (**Figure 8**).

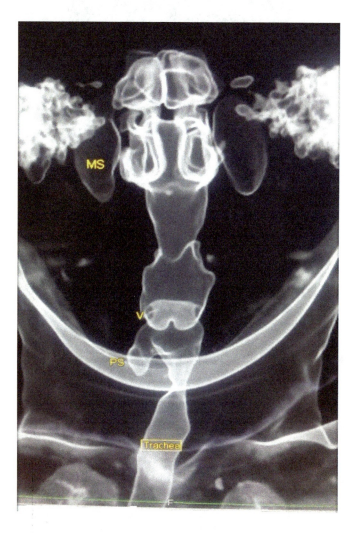

Figure 8. Antero-posterior (AP) curved MPR multi-planar reconstruction of the airway showing the entire airway in single plane from the nares down to the trachea allowing accurate measurement and orientation of the airway caliber at the different levels. **MS**: maxillary sinus; **V**: vallecula; **PS**: piriform sinus.

12. Ultrasound in airway management

12.1. Introduction

Ultrasound (US) examination of the upper airway in critically ill patients supplies a number of attractive advantages compared with competitive traditional imaging techniques or endoscopy. It is widely available, portable, repeatable, relatively cheap, pain-free, safe, and bedside machine in every operating theater and ICU suite.

12.2. Uses in airway management

- Locate the anatomy of major vessels and the thyroid gland in relation to tracheostomy site [34].

- Localize tracheal rings and cricothyroid membrane (**Figure 9**).

- Identify midline, puncture site for percutaneous tracheostomy.

- Checking of endotracheal intubation and detection of esophageal intubation [34].

- Estimation of gastric content [35].

- Recognize the air-tissue border from tongue to mid-trachea and at the pleural level [36].

- Localize the trachea by combining palpation of the sternal bone with US.

- Identify the "string of-pearls" sign that identifies the tracheal rings and mark the cricothyroid membrane as part of difficult airway management skills [34].

- Recognize sonographic evidence of lung movement during respiration and exclude a pneumothorax [34].

- Recognize endobronchial intubation and one-lung ventilation [36].

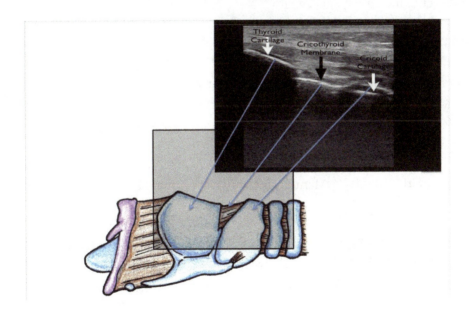

Figure 9. Ultrasound images of larynx and trachea rings.

13. Recommendations

The airway competence in ICU should be coping with the rapidly evolving advances in airway management. Therefore, efforts should be focused on the three pillars of airway mastery: airway providers as intensivists or critical care physicians, equipment, and operational plans. Not all institutions can afford all airway equipment in the market; however, they should make sure that critical care providers have a full access to the available tools and they are comfortable using it. Educational sessions and refresher courses should be tailored to meet the competence level of the ICU providers and equipment availability. Operational plan includes developing institutional airway protocols and implementing difficult airway guidelines. The protocols should consider different staffing models of ICU and make sure all the time at least one member of the team with the highest experience in airway should be always available.

14. Key points

- Airway management in intensive care patients may be lifesaving or life threatening.
- Maintenance of patent airway, adequate ventilation, and pulmonary gas exchange are very important in critically ill patients. Airway management in intensive care patients differs significantly from routine surgical procedures in the operating room.
- Critical care physicians should be familiar with the equipment and the techniques to maintain and secure the airway.

Competing interests

The authors declare that there are no competing interests.

Author details

Nabil Abdelhamid Shallik[1,2,3,4]*, Mamdouh Almustafa[5], Ahmed Zaghw[5] and Abbas Moustafa[6,7]

*Address all correspondence to: nshallik@hamad.qa

1 Hamad Medical Corporation, Clinical Anesthesiology, Weill Cornell Medical College in Qatar, Doha, Qatar

2 Anesthesia and ICU Department, Tanta Faculty of Medicine, Tanta, Egypt

3 Anesthesia Section of Rumailah Hospital, Anesthesia, ICU and Perioperative Medicine Department HMC, Doha, Qatar

4 Medical Education and Qatar Robotic Surgery Center, HMC, Doha, Qatar

5 Department of Anesthesia, ICU and Perioperative Medicine, HMC, Doha, Qatar

6 Elminia University, Egypt

7 Radiology, HMC, Doha, Qatar

References

[1] Schwartz DE, Matthay MA, Cohen NH. Death and other complications of emergency airway management in critically ill adults. Anesthesiology. 1995;**82**:367-376

[2] Jaber S, Amraoui J, Lefrant JY, Arich C, Cohendy R, Landreau L, et al. Clinical practice and risk factors for immediate complications of endotracheal intubation in the intensive care unit: A prospective, multiple-center study. Critical Care Medicine. 2006;**34**:2355-2361

[3] Adnet F, Jouriles NJ, Le Toumelin P, Hennequin B, Taillander C, Rayeh P, et al. Survey of out-of-hospital emergency intubations in the French prehospital medical system: A multicenter study. Annals of Emergency Medicine. 1998;32:454-456

[4] Griesdale DE, Bosma TL, Kurth T, Isac G, Chittock DR. Complications of endotracheal intubation in the critically ill. Intensive Care Medicine. 2008;**34**:1835-1842

[5] Tagawa T, Sakuraba S, Okuda M. Pentax-AWS-assisted insertion of a transesophageal echocardiography probe. Journal of Clinical Anesthesia. 2009;**21**(1):73-74

[6] Roberts JR, Halstead J. Passage of a nasogastric tube in an intubated patient facilitated by a video laryngoscope. The Journal of Emergency Medicine. 2011;**40**(3):330

[7] El-Tahan M, Doyle DJ, Khidr AM, Hassieb AG. Case report: Double lumen tube insertion in a morbidly obese patient through the non-channeled blade of the King Vision™ Videolaryngoscope. F1000 Research. 2014;**3**:129. DOI: 10.12688/f1000research.4481.3

[8] Kajekar P, Mendonca C, Danha R, Hillermann C. Awake tracheal intubation using Pentax airway scope in 30 patients: A case series. Indian Journal of Anaesthesia. 2014;**58**:447-451

[9] Shinohara H, Ishii H, Kakuyama M, Fukuda K. Morbidly obese patient with a huge ovarian tumor who was intubated while awake using airway scope in lateral decubitus position. Masui. 2010;**59**:625-628

[10] Hirabayashi Y, Fujita A, Seo N, Sugimoto H. A comparison of cervical spine movement during laryngoscopy using the Airtraq or Macintosh laryngoscopes. Anaesthesia. 2008;**63**(6):635-640

[11] Siu LW, Mathieson E, Naik VN, Chandra D, Joo HS. Patient- and operator-related factors associated with successful GlideScope intubations: A prospective observational study in 742 patients. Anaesthesia and Intensive Care Journal. 2010;**38**(1):70-75

[12] Maassen R, Lee R, Hermans B, Marcus M, van Zundert A. A comparison of three videolaryngoscopes: The Macintosh laryngoscope blade reduces, but does not replace, routine stylet use for intubation in morbidly obese patients. Anesthesia and Analgesia. 2009;**109**(5):1560-1565

[13] Platts-Mills TF, Campagne D, Chinnock B, Snowden B, Glickman LT, Hendey GW. A comparison of GlideScope video laryngoscopy versus direct laryngoscopy intubation in the emergency department. Academic Emergency Medicine. 2009;**16**(9):866-871

[14] Raja AS, Sullivan AF. Adoption of video laryngoscopy in Massachusetts emergency departments. The Journal of Emergency Medicine. 2012;**42**(2):233-237

[15] Diehl JL, El Atrous S, Touchard D, et al. Changes in the work of breathing induced by tracheotomy in ventilator-dependent patients. American Journal of Respiratory and Critical Care Medicine. 1999;**159**:383

[16] Lin MC, Huang CC, Yang CT, et al. Pulmonary mechanics in patients with prolonged mechanical ventilation requiring tracheostomy. Anaesthesia and Intensive Care. 1999;**27**:581

[17] Lim CK, Ruan SY, Lin FC, et al. Effect of tracheostomy on weaning parameters in difficult-to-wean mechanically ventilated patients: A prospective observational study. PLoS One. 2015;**10**:e0138294

[18] Mohr AM, Rutherford EJ, Cairns BA, Boysen PG. The role of dead space ventilation in predicting outcome of successful weaning from mechanical ventilation. The Journal of trauma. 2001;**51**:843.

[19] Fikkers BG, van Veen JA, Kooloos JG, et al. Emphysema and pneumothorax after percutaneous tracheostomy: Case reports and an anatomic study. Chest. 2004;**125**:1805.

[20] Koitschev A, Graumueller S, Zenner HP, et al. Tracheal stenosis and obliteration above the tracheostoma after percutaneous dilational tracheostomy. Critical Care Medicine. 2003;**31**:1574.

[21] Scalise P, Prunk SR, Healy D, Votto J. The incidence of tracheoarterial fistula in patients with chronic tracheostomy tubes: A retrospective study of 544 patients in a long-term care facility. Chest. 2005;**128**:3906

[22] Arola MK. Tracheostomy and its complications. A retrospective study of 794 tracheostomized patients. Annales Chirurgiae et Gynaecologiae. 1981;**70**:96

[23] Coplin WM, Pierson DJ, Cooley KD, et al. Implications of extubation delay in brain-injured patients meeting standard weaning criteria. American Journal of Respiratory and Critical Care Medicine. 2000;**161**:1530

[24] Thille AW, Boissier F, Ben Ghezala H, et al. Risk factors for and prediction by caregivers of extubation failure in ICU patients: A prospective study. Critical Care Medicine. 2015;**43**:61

[25] Nishimura M. High- flow nasal cannula oxygen therapy in adults. Journal of Intensive Care. 2015;**3**:15

[26] Patel A, Nouraei SAR. Transnasal Humidified Rapid-Insufflation Ventilatory Exchange (THRIVE): A physiological method of increasing apnoea time in patients with difficult airways. Anaesthesia. 2015;**70**:323-329

[27] Benumof JL, et al. Laryngeal mask airway and the ASA difficult airway algorithm. Anesthesiology. 1996;**84**(3);686-699

[28] Siddiqui S, Seet E, Chan WY. The use of laryngeal mask airway Supreme™ in rescue airway situation in the critical care unit. Singapore Medical Journal. 2014;**55**(12):205

[29] Brimacombe JR, Berry A. The incidence of aspiration associated with the laryngeal mask airway: A meta-analysis of published literature. Journal of Clinical Anesthesia. 1995;**7**(4):297-305

[30] Strametz R, et al. Laryngeal mask airway versus endotracheal tube for percutaneous dilatational tracheostomy in critically ill adult patients. The Cochrane Database of Systematic Reviews. 2014;**30**(6):CD009901

[31] Mort TC, Braffett BH. Conventional versus video laryngoscopy for tracheal tube exchange: Glottic visualization, success rates, complications, and rescue alternatives in the high-risk difficult airway patient. Anesthesia & Analgesia. 2015;**121**(2):440-448

[32] Finkelstein SE, Schrump DS, Nguyen DM, Hewitt SM, Kunst TF, Summers RM. Comparative evaluation of super high-resolution CT scan and virtual bronchoscopy for the detection of tracheobronchial malignancies. Chest. 2003;**124**:1834-1840

[33] Osorio F, Perilla M, Doyle DJ, Palomo JM. Cone beam computed tomography: An innovative tool for airway assessment. Anesthesia & Analgesia. 2008;**106**(6):1803-1807

[34] Drescher MJ et al. Ultrasound of Esophageal Intubation. Academic Emergency Medicine. 2000;**7**(6):722-725

[35] Perlas A, Mitsakakis N, Liu L, Cino M, Haldipur N, Davis L, Cubillos J, Chan V. Validation of a mathematical model for ultrasound assessment of gastric volume by gastroscopic examination. Anesthesia & Analgesia. 2013;**116**(2):357-363

[36] Singh M, Chin KJ, Chan VW, Wong DT, Prasad GA, Yu E. Use of sonography for airway assessment: An observational study. Journal of Ultrasound in Medicine. 2010;**29**:79-85.

Brain Death in Children

Eleni Athanasios Volakli, Peristera-Eleni Mantzafleri,
Serafeia Kalamitsou, Asimina Violaki,
Elpis Chochliourou, Menelaos Svirkos,
Athanasios Kasimis and Maria Sdougka

Abstract

Brain death (BD) is a distinct mode of death in pediatric intensive care units, accounting for 16–23% of deaths. Coma, absent brainstem reflexes, and apnea in a patient with acute irreversible neurological insult should alarm the attending physician to start the appropriate actions to establish or refute the diagnosis for BD. BD diagnosis is clinical, starting with the preconditions that should be met, and based on the examination of all brainstem reflexes, including the apnea test. Apnea testing should be conducted according to standard criteria to demonstrate the absence of spontaneous respirations, in the case of an intense ventilatory stimulus, setting at increased $PaCO_2$ levels ≥60 and ≥20 mm Hg, compared to baseline. When elements of clinical examination and/or apnea test cannot be performed, ancillary studies to demonstrate the presence/absence of electrocerebral silence and/or cerebral blood flow are guaranteed. Two clinical examinations by qualified physicians at set intervals are required. Time of death is the time of second examination and ventilator support should stop at that time, except for organ donation. The use of check list in documentation of BD helps in the uniformity of diagnosis and fosters further trust from medical, family, and community personnel.

Keywords: brain death, pediatric intensive care unit, apnea testing, brainstem reflexes, coma

1. Introduction

The evolution of intensive care has led to circumstances that a human being could be artificially maintained in life through technological advancements even in the presence of an irreversible neurological damage. Brain death (BD) in most instances occurs when an acute insult to the brain causes a neuropathologic viscious cycle of brain edema, increases intracranial pressure (ICP), and decreases cerebral blood flow that compromise blood supply to the brain and results in ischemia, a situation which resembles to "total brain infarction" according to Swedish Committee on defining death [1]. Severe traumatic head injury, infections, tumors, cerebral vascular accidents, or acute global anoxic/ischemic injury following severe respiratory failure, shock, or cardiac arrest are the main causes of BD in children [2]. Rarely, acute toxic neuronal injury as happened in fulminant hepatic failure or other metabolic diseases are the reasons, or cellular dysoxia, which prevents extraction or utilization of oxygen, as is the case in cyanide poisoning.

Brain death is a distinct mode of death both in adult and pediatric population; it is estimated that BD accounts for approximately 16–23% of deaths in the pediatric intensive care unit (PICU), while the corresponding values for adults are quite similar and depending on the nature of the unit, rising from 15% in multidisciplinary units up to 30% in neurocritical units [3–6]. Most research about BD involves adults; however, not all principles regarding BD could be transferred to children. The pediatric brain is immature; the development, plasticity, and maturation of central nervous system (CNS) ends by the 2 years of age according to the majority of researchers, while others believe to continue beyond the first decade of life [7]. Moreover, resilience to certain forms of injury could be found, due to the open fontanelles in infancy and the presence of certain forms of diseases that result in hydranencephalia and cerebral atrophy, and/or wide craniectomy, that could hasten the progress of intracranial hypertension. The above should be considered when interpreting diagnosis and confirming BD in infants and children [8].

The first effort to define BD as a new criterion for death was made in 1968 by a consensus report of the Ad Hoc Committee of the Harvard Medical School, without specific recommendations with respect to age [9]. Irreversible coma was defined as unresponsiveness to external stimuli, absent movements or breathing, absent reflexes, and a flat electroencephalograph (EEG). Later on, in 1975, on a review of the Harvard criteria by the American Academy of Neurology (AAN), they question the applicability of the consensus criteria to children stating that the above criteria may be inapplicable for children under 5 years of age since there are indications that the immature nervous system can survive significant periods of electrocerebral silence. In an effort to set a standard national definition on BD, in 1981, in the USA, the Uniform Determination of Death Act was adopted as part of the President's Commission [10]. Death was determined in accordance with accepted medical standards either as an irreversible cessation of circulatory and respiratory functions of a person, or irreversible cessation of all functions of the entire brain, including the brain stem. Age-specific guidelines were again not provided and medical standards were not described, and the commission recommended caution in applying neurological criteria to determine death in children younger than 5 years.

In 1995, the Quality Standards Subcommittee of the AAN published the practice parameters for determining brain death in adults to delineate the medical standards for the determination of BD in patients older than 18 years. The document emphasized the three cardinal clinical findings necessary to confirm irreversible cessation of all functions of the entire brain, including the brainstem: *coma or unresponsiveness* (with known cause), *absence of brainstem reflexes*, and *apnea*. Future research in apnea testing, and the need for validation of confirmatory tests was recommended [11]. However, despite the published parameters, considerable practice variations were recorded, which led to the 2010 update that sought to use evidence-based methods to answer questions historically related to variations in BD determination, to promote uniformity in diagnosis [12].

The irreversible cessations of all functions of brain, including the brainstem, are not universally accepted; the definition of BD in each nation depends on jurisdiction. In the USA, Australia, and New Zealand for example, a whole brain death definition is accepted. On the contrary, in the UK, India, and Canada a brainstem-based definition of death is in place and the term "death by neurological criteria" (DNC) is adopted [13–16]. In the UK, the most recent definition for DNC was published in 2008 by the Academy of Medical Royal Colleges (AoMRC) in the code of practice for the diagnosis and confirmation of death. Consciousness and breathing capacity were recognized as essential characteristics of life and the irreversible loss of them were regarded equal to death [13]. The applicability of the criteria in infants younger than 2 months were questioned, in agreement with a report presented by the British Paediatric Association (BPA) in 1991, which stated also that the criteria of DNC cannot be applied in infants younger than 37 weeks of gestation [17]. Caution was relieved by the guidelines issued in 2015 by the Royal College of Paediatrics and Child Health (RCCHD) considering the diagnosis of DNC in infants from 37 weeks corrected gestation (postmenstrual) to 2 months (postterm) of age. RCCHD stated that the 2008 criteria of death could be applied to this population with precautionary measures regarding the apnea test due to immaturity of the newborn infant's respiratory system [18].

The first specific pediatric guidelines on BD were issued in 1987 by the American Academy of Pediatrics (AAP) to solve questions and give answers for this special topic. These guidelines were a consensus opinion regarding necessary clinical history, physical examination criteria, observation periods, and ancillary laboratory tests required to determine brain death in children[19]. An update followed in 2011, with emphasis given to two different age populations: the one from newborn 37 weeks gestation to 30 days of life and the other from 31 days of life to 18 years [20]. These guidelines could serve as a basis for the development of national guidelines at each nation, taking into account legal, cultural, and religious differences, and will be analyzed in this chapter, enriched by the experience of a single centre and the discussion of relevant references.

BD in most occasions is intertwined to organ harvesting and transplantation, and much research in the field has been done through national organ procurement databases [21, 22]. Nevertheless, the declaration of BD should be done by the patient physicians only, according to local national and institutional guidelines, irrespective from the transplantation team [23, 24]. The priority of the medical system is to save lives rather than to obtain organs and the public must feel confident that they would become organ donors only after all reasonable attempts to save their lives have failed. Maintenance of public trust is essential for the functioning of organ transplantation systems around the world [24]. BD is still a controversial issue for some physicians, and civilians as well, who deny the conceptual basis for equating an irreversibly nonfunctioning brain with a dead human being [25]. Though, the ethical, psychosocial, and philosophical approach of BD is beyond the scope of this chapter which will concentrate on the biological and clinical approach only of pediatric patients dying from BD.

2. Dying from BD in the PICU

Regardless some terminology differences between the most widely USA definition of BD as the death of the whole brain, and the UK definition of death by DNC as the death of the brainstem, the concept that is universally accepted is that *the patient dying from BD suffered an acute irreversible CNS insult that resulted to coma, absent brainstem reflexes, and apnea* [7]. Although cases of confirmation of BD in children have been described outside the PICU, the proper place where the patients should be treated and diagnosis takes place is the PICU [22–24]. Frequently, the first indication by the bedside nurse is the lack of spontaneous awakening periods, the absence of cough during suctioning, and the fixed dilated pupils, which should alarm the attending physician that the patient deteriorates, and may be is going to BD. All sedative medications, including antiepileptic drugs and neuromuscular blocking agents, should stop at that time, the patient should continue to receive the maximum supportive intensive care treatment to preserve homeostasis, and the preparations should begin to establish or refute the diagnosis of BD. The diagnosis of BD is confirmed by clinical examination criteria only, based on the absence of neurologic function with a known irreversible cause of coma. Ancillary studies are not required except in cases where the clinical examination and apnea test cannot be completed [13, 14, 20].

3. Management of critically ill children dying from BD

For the better understanding of the evolution to BD in children, we will present the sequence of the events that happen in pediatric patients treated in a PICU after a severe neurological insult, step by step, in a timely manner. Our data were obtained from a retrospective study regarding all deaths that occurred between January 2011 and April 2016, in a multidisciplinary eight-bed PICU of Northern Greece. Among 275 deaths, 44 (16%) were defined as BD. The incidence was higher in boys (28/44 patients, 63.6%). Mean age was 68.75 ± 44.04 months (range 2 months to 13 years) and mean severity of illness as estimated with the pediatric risk of mortality (PRISM III-24 h) score at admission was 21.67 ± 9.98. Head injury was the most frequent cause of BD (29.41%) followed by CNS infection (23.52%), hypoxic/ischemic insults (23.52%), CNS tumors (11.76%), and intracranial bleeding (11.76%).

The management of the patients was done under the relevant for the diagnosis international protocols, under sedation, mechanical ventilation, chemoprophylaxis, gastric ulcer prophylaxis, and artificial nutrition. At admission, 88.6% of patients were already on mechanical ventilation and almost half of them (52.3%) were in shock. Central venous catheters and arterial lines were inserted in all patients. Nine patients (20.5%) had intracranial pressure (ICP) monitoring. Almost all received osmotherapy with either NaCl 3% (37 patients, 84.1%) and/or mannitol 20% (36 patients, 81.8%). Sedation was achieved with midazolam at mean max dose of 0.93 ± 0.56 mg/kg/h and remifantanil at max dose of 0.09 ± 0.05 mcg/kg/min. Cis-attracurium was administered for neuromuscular blocking at a bolus dose of 0.2 mg/kg, as needed before interventions, e.g., suctioning to avoid inadvertent increase in ICP. Sodium thiopental at a max dose of 5 mg/kg/h was administered in 18 patients (40.9%) and four patients (9.1%) were treated with craniectomy, as a third tier therapy to refractory intracranial hypertention [26]. Diabetes insipidus was recorded in 33 patients (75%), and high sugar levels needed insulin therapy in 19 patients (43.2%). The higher serum Na and sugar levels that were recorded were 165 ± 15.39 mmol/l and 281 ± 159.07 mg/dl, respectively. During their stay, the majority of the patients (79.5%) needed inotropic and/or vasopressor support to preserve an acceptable hemodynamic status.

The clinical suspicion on BD was set on 3.59 ± 5.46 day through dilated unreacted pupils. Mean pupil size at admission was 4.07 ± 2.06 mm which was increased to the final size of 6.28 ± 1.13 mm. Following that all the prerequisites of BD were fulfilled, two clinical examinations were performed by a panel of three doctors registered for at least 2 years; one anesthetist, one neurologist or neurosurgeon, and the attending physician (pediatrician or pediatric surgeon), according to the Greek law. Mean sedation time was 4.02 ± 3.03 days. The first tests were done in 9.88 ± 6.50 days after admission and the second in 11.28 ± 6.53 days. Mean time between tests was 27.54 ± 11.80 h. Apnea testing was prepared according to national BD protocol, with preoxygenation with 100% oxygen for at least 10 min, and baseline mechanical ventilation aimed at 40 mmHg of $PaCO_2$ [11]. Oxygenation during apnea was done through a catheter tailored to endotracheal tube (ETT) size (size in CH doubled the ID size of ETT in mm), inserted in the endotracheal tube at a length corresponded to tracheal carina, with a flow of 1 l/min/age in years, initially, according to acute pediatric life support (APLS) recommendation for apneic oxygenation [27]. If oxygenation was inadequate, a gradually increase in O_2 flow in increments of 1 l/min up to max 12 l/min was performed [12]. For this purpose, we used a simple suction catheter of appropriate size as described above, with the valve occluded, and connected to an oxygen flow source, preferably a low pressure one (capable of giving oxygen at driving pressure of 1–2 bar). In the case of acute respiratory distress syndrome (ARDS), hypoxia, and need for high positive end expiratory pressure (PEEP), apnea testing was performed on continuous positive airway pressure (CPAP) modality. Duration of apnea was 10 min if feasible, or earlier if signs of hypoxia and/or hypotension appeared. Apnea testing was considered positive for BD if no spontaneous respiration occurred when the $PaCO_2$ level was >60 and >20 mmHg compared to baseline, in accordance with international guidelines [11, 12, 14].

A total of 88 apnea tests were recorded. Incomplete data concerning the way of oxygenation during the apnea test were revealed in 50% of the tests, probably due to the retrospective data analysis and incomplete recordings. Thirty-six patients (81.81%) completed the test successfully. Eleven apnea tests (12.5%) were aborted, mainly due to hypoxia (8/11, 72.72%) and to a lesser degree due to shock (3/11, 27.27%). In detail, four patients did not manage to complete the first apnea test (three hypoxia, one shock), while seven patients aborted the second test (five hypoxia, two shock). The data of apnea testing are presented in **Table 1**. Ancillary study with magnetic resonance angiography (MRA) was carried out in eight patients (18.18%). Patients died 54.58 ± 59.64 h after the completion of the second apnea test. Three families (6.81%) gave consent for organ donation.

	Mechanical ventilation mode	FiO$_2$%	pH	PaO$_2$ (mmHg)	PaCO$_2$ (mmHg)
Baseline	IPPV (68.4%)	50.8 ± 20.6	7.44 ± 0.062	133.88 ± 33.90	33.36 ± 4.60
	PRVC (22.5%)				
	SIMV-PS (9.1%)				
A. prep.		100	7.33 ± 0.084	382 ± 97.59	45.46 ± 4.18
A. Apnea test	CPAP (20.4%)	100	7.10 ± 0.063	235 ± 107.18	84.15 ± 10.53
	Tracheal O$_2$ (29.6%)				
	NA (50%)				
B. Prep.		100	7.33 ± 0.073	354 ± 127	45.21 ± 5.20
B. Apnea test	CPAP (22.7%)	100	7.11 ± 0.063	223 ± 129.72	84.79 ± 13.99
	Tracheal O$_2$ (25%)				
	NA (52.3%)				

IPPV, intermittent postitive pressure ventilation; PRVC, pressure regulated volume control; SIMV-PS, synchronized intermittend mandatory ventilation-pressure support; CPAP, continuous positive airway pressure; Tracheal O$_2$, tracheal insufflation of oxygen at age-related flows of 1 l/min/age (max 12 l/min); NA, not applicable (lack of data).

Table 1. Data of apnea testing ($n = 77$) in pediatric BD patients ($n = 44$).

4. Guidelines for the determination of BD in infants and children

4.1. Definition of BD

In 2011, a multidisciplinary committee was formed by the Society of Critical Care Medicine (SCCM) and the AAP to update the 1987 Task Force Recommendations for the diagnosis of pediatric BD [12, 14, 20]. According to guidelines, *BD is a clinical diagnosis based on the absence of neurologic function with a known diagnosis that has resulted in irreversible coma.* Coma and apnea must coexist to diagnose DB. A complete neurologic examination is mandatory to determine BD with all components appropriately documented. An algorithm for the diagnosis of BD in children adapted from Ref. [20] is provided in Appendix 1.

4.2. Age definition

Two age definitions were set with an impact on the timing of first exam and the observation period between tests.

- Newborns 37 weeks gestation to 30 days of life.
- Infants 31 days of life to 18 years.

Because of insufficient data in the literature, recommendations for preterm infants less than 37 weeks gestational age were not included in this guideline.

4.3. Timing of first exam

- Twenty-four hours for patients aged from 37 weeks gestation to 30 days of life. Time is counted after birth, cardiac arrest with successful resuscitation or other severe neurological insult.

- Twelve hours for patients aged 31 days of life to 18 years. Time is counted after cardiac arrest with successful resuscitation or other severe neurological insult.

It is reasonable to defer neurologic examination to determine brain death for longer than 24 h, if dictated by clinical judgment of the treating physician. Neonates who probably suffered from hypoxic/ischemic insult during the neonatal period and had been put in therapeutic hypothermia deserve a longer observation time before the first examination. Hypothermia not only could interfere with brainstem reflexes interpretation but hastens drug metabolism as well. In addition, the first examination should be postponed beyond 24 h if residual drug effect is suspected. In general, the first examination cannot be performed unless all the preconditions of diagnosing BD are met.

4.4. Irreversible and identifiable cause of coma

A known and irreversible cause of coma should be established before the diagnosis of BD. In most instances, the evolution of a brain damage to BD is depicted with computed tomography (CT) or magnetic resonance imaging (MRI). Sometimes, neuroimaging if performed early enough in the course of the disease is without significant findings. Serial examinations in such occasions are helpful. CT and MRI are introductory studies and should not be relied on to make the determination of brain death. Additional data such as results from cerebrospinal fluid (CSF) analysis and/or other microbiological data are supportive [12]. In 2011 AAP guidelines, three major causes of coma were recognized: traumatic brain injury, anoxic brain injury, and known metabolic disorder. In cases that the cause of coma is not identifiable, the physician should specify the cause of coma as "Other." It is advisable to keep these major causes when recording BD, which will enable international comparisons, if needed.

4.5. Preconditions

The interpretation and validity of the clinical neurological examination and the apnea testing should not leave any space for concern. All the potentially influencing factors must be corrected in advance and the subsequent undeniable preconditions must be met:

- *Cardiovascular stability.* Mean or arterial systolic pressure should be normal for age (no less than two standard deviations from the mean age responding values). Inotropic and vasomotor support may be necessary for the treatment of shock. Direct arterial pressure measurement is strongly recommended, not only for the monitoring but for blood gases analysis and $PaCO_2$ evaluation as well, which is an integral part of the apnea testing that follow.

- *Normothermia.* Therapeutic hypothermia is increasingly used as an adjunctive therapy of the insulted brain and the physician should be aware of the potential hypothermia impact on the diagnosis of brain death. Hypothermia is a depressant to central nervous system activity and may lead to a false diagnosis of brain death. Metabolism and clearance of medications are retarded, which can interfere with brain death examination. Achieving normothermia with a core body temperature of 35°C (95°F) before the first exam and maintaining it throughout the observation period is essential.

- *Homeostasis.* The most common metabolic disturbance during BD is hypernatremia due to diabetes insipidus that should be corrected with the administration of antidiouretic hormone or desmopressin. Hyperglygemia is common too, and close monitoring of glucose levels and treatment with insulin when necessary is indicated. Hyponatremia, hypoglycemia, hypothyroidism, severe pH disturbances, severe hepatic or renal dysfunction or inborn errors of metabolism may also occur and cause a potentially reversible coma in pediatric patients. All the above should be excluded before moving on diagnostic tests for BD. A high index of clinical suspicion for metabolic disturbances should be especially raised in situations where the clinical history alone does not provide a reasonable explanation for the evolution of BD.

- *Neuromuscular blocking (NMB) agents.* Adequate clearance of these agents should be confirmed. In case there is a doubt for residual NMB action, a nerve stimulator with documentation of neuromuscular junction activity and twitch response should be used to demonstrate good neuromuscular activity with 4/4 responds in "train of four" testing [12, 23].

- *Drug intoxications.* Barbiturates, opioids, sedative and anesthetic agents, antiepileptic agents, and alcohols should be discontinued. Adequate clearance (based on the age of the child, presence of organ dysfunction, total amount of medication administered, elimination half-life of the drug and any active metabolites) should be allowed before the neurologic examination. Recommendations of time intervals before brain death evaluation for many of the commonly used medications administered to critically ill neonates and children are listed in Appendix 2 of 2011 AAP guidelines. Laboratory testing of drug levels should be performed if there is a concern regarding residual drug effect. Although there is evidence that therapeutic and subtherapeutic barbiturate levels (phenobarbital and pentobarbital at 15–40 ug/ml) did not interfere with the reliability of BD diagnosis, it is advised these drugs to be at the low to mid therapeutic range before neurological examination [28]. Unusual causes of coma such as neurotoxins and chemical exposure, e.g., organophosphates and carbamates, should be occluded in rare cases where an etiology for coma has not been established.

4.6. Physical examination: coma

The neurologic examination BD criteria in pediatrics have been adapted from 2010 American Academy of Neurology criteria for BD determination in adults [12]. Patients must exhibit complete loss of consciousness, vocalization, and volitional activity and should be in a profound state of coma. Flaccid tone is confirmed by passive range of motion in extremities given there are no limitations to performing such an examination, e.g., previous trauma, and the patient is observed for any spontaneous or induced movements. Noxious stimuli in the cranial nerve distribution (deep supraorbital and/or condylomandibular pressure) and all four limbs (deep bed nail pressure), and trunk (sternal rub) should be applied and the responses, if any, should be carefully evaluated. Central (in the territory of cranial nerves, e.g., facial area) responsiveness to central and peripheral (outside the territory of cranial nerves) noxious stimuli must be absent, apart from spinally mediated reflexes. Complete absence of motion would equate a Glasgow Coma Scale (GCS) of 3. Observations such as decerebrate or decorticate posturing, true extensor or flexor motor responses to painful stimuli and seizures are not compatible with BD. Any motor response within the cranial nerve distribution, or any response in the limbs in response to cranial nerve stimulation, *precludes determination of brain death*. Spinal reflexes should be suspected in cases of motor responses in a somatic distribution after noncranial, e.g., peripheral nerve stimulus and not after stimulus in the cranial nerve territory [14].

4.7. Brainstem reflexes

The absence of all brain stem reflexes must be confirmed by the physical examination. Afferent and efferent pathways of cranial nerves are given in parentheses:

- *Oculomotor reflex (afferent II, efferent III)*. Pupils must be >4mm up to 9 mm with absent pupillary response to bright light in both eyes. Fixed midsized or fully dilated pupils are common. In cases of uncertainty, a magnifying glass could be used. Interpret with caution pupil size less than 4 mm. Small constricted pupils should be suspected for drug intoxication [12, 14].

- *Corneal reflex (afferent V, efferent VII)*. Special care should be taken not to damage the cornea during the examination. The absence of eyelid movements must be documented after touching the cornea with a cotton swab, a piece of gauze, paper, or water squirts.

- *Absence of facial or bulbar musculature movement in noxious stimulus (afferent V, efferent VII)*. Deep pressure on the condyles at the level of the temporomandibular joints and deep pressure at the supraorbital ridge should produce no grimacing or facial muscle movement.

- *Oculovestibular reflex (caloric reflex, afferent VIII, efferent III, VI)*. Check for patency of the external auditory canal with otoscopic examination. The eardrum should be visible, or it should be cleared before the test. Oculovestibular reflex is tested by irrigating each ear with ice water (caloric testing) after the head is elevated to 30° to place the horizontal semicircular canal in a horizontal position [14]. Each external auditory canal is irrigated (one ear at a time) with >10–50 ml of ice water. Movement of the eyes should be absent during 1 min of observation. Both sides are tested, with an interval of several minutes.

- *Oculocephalic reflex (eye doll reflex)*. The same pathways as in the case of oculovestibular reflex are tested. Not required any more in AAP 2011 and ANZICS 2013 guidelines due to the fact that it is not considered strong enough stimuli to elicit a response and the risk of exacerbating possible cervical spinal trauma [14].

- *Gag reflex (afferent IX, efferent X).* The pharyngeal or gag reflex is tested after stimulation of the posterior pharynx using a tongue blade or suction device. The sucking and rooting reflexes are sought in neonates and infants [20].

- *Cough—tracheal reflex (afferent X).* The tracheal reflex is most reliably tested by examining the cough response to tracheal suctioning. The catheter should be inserted into the trachea and advanced to the level of the carina followed by one or two suctioning passes. The efferent limbs for this reflex are the phrenic nerve and the thoracic and abdominal musculature. Therefore, it cannot be assessed in patients with high cervical cord injury [12].

4.8. Apnea test

Only if all the above reflexes are absent, proceed with testing for apnea. The apnea test should be conducted last so that a high $PaCO_2$ does not confound the testing of the other cranial nerves [14]. Apnea testing is the cornerstone for the diagnosis of BD both in adults and children and is conducted similar to adults. However, despite the consensus criteria published for adults and pediatrics, considerable variation has been described in performing the apnea test in both populations [2, 21, 22, 29]. In 1987 Task Force guidelines for pediatric BD is reported that apnea testing using standardized methods can be performed, but this is ordinarily done only after other examination criteria are met. Yet, the standardized methods are not described and the two associated references reported different ways of performing the apnea test. The former, by Outwaker and Rockoff, described apnea testing in 10 children aged 10 months to 13 years who met the conventional criteria for BD. In their study, oxygen 100% was provided for 5 min before the test, the ventilator rate was set to zero, and a continuous flow of oxygen was provided through the ETT. Arterial blood gases (ABG) were drawn at 0, 1, 2, 3, and 5 min. All patients completed the test successfully; mean $PaCO_2$ was 39.4 ± 7.4 mm Hg at the beginning and 59.5 ± 10.2 at the end of the test, with a mean rise of 4.0 ± 0.9 mm Hg/min [30]. The latter, by Rowland and coworkers, in 9 children aged 4 months to 13 years, mentioned that PCO_2 rise was faster than adults, and faster in the beginning of apnea test (4.4 ± 1.6, 3.4 ± 1.3 and 2.6 ± 1.2 mm Hg/min at 5, 10, and 15 min, respectively). $PaCO_2$ ranged from 60 to 116 mm Hg after 15 min of apnea. All apnea tests were accomplished uneventfully and no spontaneous respirations were observed in any of the patients after 15 min of apnea. The authors recommended that prevention of hypoxia can be reliably achieved with administration of 100% oxygen for 10 min before discontinuing ventilator support, and continuing oxygen (6 l/min) through a catheter into the length of the ETT for the duration of the test. An initial apnea test of 10 min was proposed, and if the desired levels of PCO_2 failed to achieve, then a repeated test with a longer duration of 15 min was advised. The study concluded that apneic oxygenation can be safely conducted in children as a component of the clinical evaluation of BD [31].

The above studies performed apnea testing differently. Even in the recent guidelines, there are no accurate instructions on how to perform a safe apnea test in children. Questions such as how much time is necessary for the preoxygenation period, which is the optimum baseline PCO_2 level, which is the best way for apneic oxygenation, how to prevent hypoxia and/or hypotention during the apnea test, which is the exact duration of apnea testing, remain blurred and left to the resolution of the attending physician. Physicians should always remember that *apnea testing is the last element in clinical diagnosis of BD in suspected BD children*. There are references of prospective, retrospective studies, and case reports, in suspected BD children, mentioning that occasionally patients developed spontaneous breathing during apnea testing [2, 32–35]. These references not at all blunt the validity of apnea; on the contrary they confirm the value of the test on establishing pediatric BD. Not all parts of pediatric brain die simultaneously, especially in patients with preexisting neurologic disease. In cases that apnea is not positive for BD the patient is returned back to full support, until a following apnea test can be performed or an auxiliary test is pursued to establish or refute the diagnosis. It is worth mentioning that almost in all the aforementioned reports, most children died ultimately shortly afterwards, by a second apnea test that confirmed BD diagnosis or spontaneous cardiac arrest. One patient, who never fulfilled apnea testing, and therefore BD, remained in severe neurological impairment, keeping in life technology dependent, through tracheostomy, home mechanical ventilation, and gastrostomy [34]. Brain recovery of children that met all adult BD criteria based on neurologic examination has not been confirmed so far. The apparent reversibility of brain death reported by some authors through spontaneous respirations during apnea testing is questionable; further review of these cases would reveal that those children could not had fulfilled strict brain death criteria by currently accepted medical standards. There is no documented case of a person who *fulfils the preconditions and criteria for brain death* ever subsequently developing any return of brain function [8, 14, 18, 20, 23].

4.9. Performing apnea testing

The rationale behind the apnea test is that an intense ventilator stimulus, such as hypercapnia/respiratory acidosis is needed, to stimulate respiratory drive centers in the medulla to start respiratory efforts. During this procedure, concomitant hypoxemia should be avoided by the administration of 100% O_2. The levels of PCO_2 sufficient to stimulate the respiratory drive (PCO_2 threshold) was set at 60 mm Hg, based on the study of Scafer and Caronna, which report that three comatose, apparently BD adults, started to breath at PCO_2 levels of 44–56 mmHg [36]. According to AAP 2011 guidelines, if no respiratory effort is observed from the initiation of the apnea test to the time the measured $PaCO_2$ is ≥60 and ≥20 mm Hg above the baseline, the apnea test is consistent with brain death. Patients with chronic respiratory disease and chronic hypercapnia may need a higher respiratory stimulus, and in this case, the limit of ≥20 mm Hg above baseline is more appropriate.

Apnea testing should not pose risk in the patients tested; it should be safe, accurate, and reproducible [29]. In the literature, there is evidence that approximately 10% of all apnea tests are aborted (12.5% in our study), mainly due to hypoxia and to a lesser degree due to hypotension [22]. A preparation period is necessary; a fluid bolus, e.g., R/L 20 ml/kg (iv), may be helpful in the case of volume depletion in the context of diabetes insipidus that may be present; and inotropes and vasopressors should be ready and connected in line, even if they are not needed before apnea testing. The effects of raised PCO_2 levels in the circulatory system can vary. There could be an increase in heart rate and blood pressure due to sympathetic stimulation, or blood pressure may start falling due to the vasodilatation caused by the rising

PCO_2 levels and the myocardial depression caused by the acidosis; arterial line is necessary for a beat to beat evaluation of blood pressure and drug titration. Oxygenation is mostly maintained by the preoxygenation with 100% O_2 for 10 min, and through the apneic oxygenation during the test with the oxygen-diffusion technique, e.g., with tracheal insufflation of oxygen at a rate suitable for the age of the child (as described previously in our study). The catheter administrating oxygen should not be cut, the size should be appropriate to permit escaping for the excess oxygen through the ETT and prevent air trapping, and the oxygen rate should be appropriate; if these precautions are not met, there is a risk for inadvertent high oxygen pressures. Cases of barotrauma with pneumothoraces and/or pneumomediastinum have been described during apnea testing and should be avoided [37, 38]. In the case of hypoxia, CPAP could be applied through the application of the suitable valve in the T-piece. A Mapleson anesthesia bag attached to the ETT could also be used. There are reports of successfully performing the apnea test through a T-piece attached to the ET only; however, a question is arising if oxygen flowing simply at the end of ETT is capable of reaching the trachea to diffuse in the alveoli. Accomplishing apnea testing with the patient connected to ventilator should be avoided because all modern ventilators have built in apnea back up modes that do not allow zeroing the respiratory rate for a long time. Moreover, cardiac beating could trigger the ventilator if strong enough, and a false indication of spontaneous respiratory effort may appear. Maintenance of the homeostasis is of paramount importance for the safe and successful performance of the apnea test:

- Regular arterial blood gas (ABG) analysis should ensure normalization of the pH and $PaCO_2$; maintenance of core temperature above 35°C and normotension for age should be confirmed, even through dose adjustment of inotropic and vasopressor agents. Still in hemodynamic stable patients before the test, these drugs should be ready and connected to line for immediate hemodynamic support, in case hypotension occurs.

- Preoxygenation using 100% oxygen, aiming at nitrogen removal and oxygen enrichment, should be applied for at least 10 min [12]. Mechanical ventilation parameters could be modified as well at the same time, it is advisable to keep tidal volume and PEEP at the same level to avoid derecruitment and decrease only the respiratory rate aimed at eucapnia with baseline PCO_2 level of 35–45 mm Hg. This could facilitate the rise in $PaCO_2$ to the desired levels for a positive apnea testing [11, 12, 14].

- Intermittent mandatory mechanical ventilation is discontinued once the patient is well oxygenated and a normal $PaCO_2$ around 40 mm Hg has been achieved. Oxygenation should be accomplished with the apneic oxygenation method through the ETT as described earlier. The patient could also be changed to a T-piece attached to the ETT, or a self-inflating bag such as a Mapleson circuit connected to the ETT, or CPAP in cases of hypoxemia.

- Cardiac beating, blood pressure, and oxygen saturation should be continuously monitored while observing carefully for spontaneous respiratory effort (any respiratory muscle activity that results in abdominal or chest excursions or activity of accessory respiratory muscles) throughout the entire procedure [14].

- If the patient is well oxygenated ($SpO_2 > 85\%$) and hemodynamic stable, keep apnea duration to 10 min and then draw ABG for analysis. The longer the apnea times the more the possibilities for a positive apnea test. AAP 2011 guidelines suggest serial follow up ABG to monitor the rise in $PaCO_2$ while the patient remains disconnected from mechanical ventilation [20].

- Apnea test is consistent with brain death if no respiratory effort is observed for 10 min or the time (if earlier) that values of measured $PaCO_2$ ≥60 and ≥20 mm Hg above the baseline level are achieved. The patient should be placed back on mechanical ventilator support and medical management should continue until the confirmation of BD is completed by the second neurologic examination and the second apnea test.

- If oxygen saturations fall below 85% or hemodynamic instability limits completion of apnea testing draw ABG at this time, discontinue the test and return the patient to ventilator and full support. If $PaCO_2$ level of ≥60 and ≥20 mm Hg above the baseline has not been achieved at that time, another attempt to test for apnea may be performed at a later time, or an ancillary study may be pursued to assist with determination of brain death.

- Observation of any respiratory effort is inconsistent with brain death and the apnea test should be aborted.

- Use of a capnograph to detect spontaneous respirations through end tidal $EtCO_2$ fluctuations is desirable.

4.10. Inability to perform elements of clinical examination and/or apnea

Clinical neurological examination and/or apnea test cannot be performed under some circumstances, especially during trauma. Ocular trauma, severe maxilofascial injuries, skull base fractures that are running through the external ear canal, and ear drum rupture limit the ability to perform and evaluate many of the brainstem reflexes. Cervical spinal trauma with possible participation of phrenic nerve limits the spontaneous breathing ability during apnea testing. Flaccid tone in patients with high spinal cord injury or neuromuscular diseases poses further concerns about the validity of clinical examination.

Furthermore, apnea testing cannot be performed in cases of severe hypoxia, e.g., in ARDS patients even under CPAP conditions, and/or in patients with severe hemodynamic instability. When concerns about the potentials and validity of elements of clinical examination and/or apnea testing are arisen, then continued observation is recommended. A valid neurologic evaluation and apnea test could be performed at a later time, as soon as all issues are resolved. If this is not possible, then an ancillary study is indicated to establish BD diagnosis.

4.11. Ancillary studies

The 2011 AAP BD guidelines recommends that ancillary studies (electroencephalogram and radionuclide cerebral blood flow) are not required to establish brain death and are not a substitute for the neurologic examination. The term "ancillary study" is preferred to "confirmatory study" since these tests assist the clinician in making the clinical diagnosis of brain death. Ancillary studies are not common in places where the DNC concept, as the death of the brainstem, is accepted; on the contrary they are more common where the whole concept of BD, including the death of the brainstem, is acknowledged. Nevertheless, apart the above mentioned reasons that question the potential and safety of clinical examination, ancillary studies are sought also in suspected drug intoxication and to reduce the inter-examination observation period.

Before the use of ancillary studies, all the preconditions of BD that could be applied, and all parts of clinical examination, including apnea test, that could be performed, should be recorded. When an ancillary study supports the diagnosis of BD, a second clinical examination and apnea test must be done and components that can be completed must remain consistent with brain death. In this instance, the inter-examination observation interval may be shortened and the second clinical evaluation and apnea test (or all components that can be completed safely) can be performed and documented at any time thereafter for children of all ages [20].

4.11.1. EEG

Electroencephalograph (EEG) has been extensively studied in 485 suspected BD pediatric patients where signs of electrocerebral silence (ECS) were sought. In their first study, 76% of patients had ECS, which elevated to 89% in subsequent, if any, studies. Sixty-six patients had a second study that confirmed the ECS of the first study in 64/66 patients (97%). The two patients who showed EEG activity, in retrospect in depth analysis, would not have met the recent criteria for BD due to pharmacological agents present at the time of examination (a newborn with high phenobarbital levels of 30 μg/ml and a 5 years head trauma boy that received pentobarbital and pancuronium at the time of testing). In case that the first study showed EEG activity (85 patients), the second study showed ECS in 47/85 (55%) of patients. The rest 38/45 patients (45%), either did not have a second examination, or an ECG activity, as expected, were confirmed. It is worth mentioning that all the examined patients died (spontaneously or by withdrawal of support). Only one patient survived with severe neurological impairment from this entire group of 485 patients, the above-mentioned neonate with an elevated phenobarbital level, whose first EEG showed photic response [20].

4.11.2. CBF

Four-vessel cerebral angiography is the gold standard for determining the absence of cerebral blood flow (CBF). However, the technique is not always available, is very invasive and difficult to perform in young infants, and carry all the risk of transferring a potentially unstable patient outside the PICU. Thus, use of radionuclide CBF determinations to document the absence of CBF, with portable scanners where feasible, remains the most widely used methods to support the clinical diagnosis of brain death in infants and children. Evidence suggests that radionuclide CBF study can be used in patients with high dose barbiturate or other drugs therapy to demonstrate the absence of CBF. The classical appearance in a CBF scanning study positive for BD is the "hollow skull phenomenon" or "hot nose sign" due to the absence of circulation in the brain with relatively increased nasal region perfusion due to preserved external carotid artery flow [12, 20].

An extended study of CBF in 681 suspected BD patients showed that 86% of patients who met clinical BD criteria had absent CBF on first examination, a percentage that rose to 89% in case they had a following test. Among them, 26 patients had a second examination that confirm the absence of CBF in 24/26 patients (92%). The two exceptions with no flow in the first study that revealed some flow in the second study were two newborns. The first newborn had minimal flow on the second study and ventilator support was discontinued. The other newborn developed flow on the second study and had some spontaneous respirations and activity, and survived with severe neurologic impairment. Along with the 34 patients that had present flow in first study, 9/34 (26%) had no flow on the subsequent study, due to evolution to BD. The remaining 25/34 (74%) either had preserved flow or no further CBF studies were done, and all died (either spontaneously or by withdrawal of support). Interestingly, only one patient survived from this entire group (the one mentioned earlier) with severe neurologic deficit [20].

4.11.3. ECG versus CBF

There are 12 studies in the literature examining 149 suspected BD patients of any age with both initial EEG and CBF studies, which present special interest to compare one to another for their diagnostic yield. Data were stratified by three age groups: (i) all children ($n = 149$); (ii) newborns (<1 month of age, $n = 30$); and (iii) children aged >1 month to 18 years ($n = 119$). In the first EEG study, ECS was found in 70% in the whole cohort, 40% in newborns and 78% in older children. Similarly, the absence of flow in the first CBF study was documented in the same proportion in all age groups (70%), though performance was better in infants with absent flow in 63%, whereas in older children remained the same with absent flow in 71% of patients. Both studies were compatible with BD in 58% of all patients, only in 26% of newborns and 66% of older children. It seemed that for newborns, EEG with ECS was less sensitive (40%) than the absence of CBF (63%) when confirming the diagnosis of brain death, but even in the CBF group the yield was low. Performance was better for children older than 1 month of age and both of these ancillary studies remain accepted tests to assist with determination of brain death and are of similar confirmatory value. Radionuclide CBF techniques are increasingly being used in many institutions replacing EEG [20].

If the results of the ancillary study are equivocal, the patient cannot be pronounced BD. Observation under maximum supportive care is continued until a valid clinical examination and apnea testing is possible, or a subsequent ancillary study with definite results can be performed. A waiting period of 24 h is recommended before further radionuclide CBF study is performed, to allow for adequate clearance of Tc-99m. A waiting period of 24 h is reasonable and recommended before repeating EEG ancillary study as well.

There are reports of other newer ancillary studies performed in adults and children with suspected BD. Concerning the adult population, Transcranial Doppler is not included in adult AAN 2010 guidelines, whereas it is reported as a screening only test in ANZICS 2013 guidelines [12,14]. MRA angiography, CT angiography, somatosensory evoked potentials, and bispectral index are mentioned in adult 2010 guidelines but are not recommended due to insufficient evidence [12]. Correspondingly, pediatric AAP 2011 guidelines cannot recommend any of the above studies as ancillary studies to assist with the determination of BD in children [20].

4.12. Number of examinations

Two examinations, including apnea testing with each examination, separated by an observation period, are required. The examinations should be performed by different attending physicians involved in the care of the child, or as specified by national law. The first examination determines the child has met neurologic examination criteria for brain death. The second examination, performed by a different attending physician, confirms brain death, based on an unchanged and irreversible condition.

4.13. Number of examiners

According to AAP 2011 guidelines, two physicians (one each time) must perform two independent examinations separated by specific intervals. Apnea testing, as an objective test, could be performed by the same physician, preferably the attending physician who is managing ventilator care of the child. The committee recommends that these examinations be performed by different attending physicians involved in the care of the child. Physicians should have experience with neonates, infants, and children and have specific training in neurocritical care. They must be competent to perform the clinical examination and interpret results from ancillary studies. Pediatric intensivists and neonatologists, pediatric neurologists and neurosurgeons, pediatric trauma surgeons, and pediatric anesthesiologists with critical care training could serve as examiners for BD diagnosis in children. Adult specialists should have the appropriate neurologic and critical care training to diagnose brain death in children. Junior doctors, residents, and fellows should be encouraged to learn how to properly perform brain death testing by observing and participating in BD diagnosis performed by senior experienced attending physicians.

The exact number, specialty, and the required qualifications of the examiners vary according to national law; e.g., in Greece, three physicians (anesthetist, neurologist/neurosurgeon, and attending physician such as pediatrician/pediatric surgeon), who should be board registered for their specialty at least for 2 years, are required. The same panel of doctors is mandatory to perform the second examination at the set observation period. No one must be potentially involved in the organ donation and transplantation team.

4.14. Observation period

The recommended observation periods are as follows:

- 24 h for neonates (37 weeks gestation to term infants 30 days of age).
- 12 h for infants and children (>30 days to 18 years).

Observation period could be shortened in case of an ancillary study compatible with BD. On this occasion, the second neurologic examination and apnea test (or all components that can be completed safely) can be performed and documented at any time thereafter for children of all ages [20].

5. Special considerations for term newborns (37 weeks gestation to 30 days of age) by AAP 2011 guidelines

The younger the patient the greater the challenge of diagnosing BD in pediatric patients; the younger the patient the longer the observation period, unless clinical BD diagnosis is supported with ancillary studies whereas the observation period could be shortened [20]. Interestingly, the performances of ancillary studies which are supposed to help in the diagnosis are less accurate in very young infants. These reservations were recorded for the first time in AAP 1987 guidelines and are listed below for historical reasons [19]. Different diagnostic criteria were defined in those guidelines according three age categories starting from the 7th day of life; no recommendation was done then for neonates younger than 7 days of life due to insufficient data. Ancillary studies, especially EEG, were regarded an essential component of the diagnosis and were mandatory with different observation periods across age:

- Infants 7 days to 2 months: Two examinations and two EEG separated by at least 48 h.

- Children 2 months to 1 year: Two examinations and two EEG separated by at least 24 h. The second EEG was not necessary if a concomitant cerebral radionuclide scan or cerebral angiography demonstrated no flow or visualization of the cerebral arteries.

- Children older than 1 year: A shorter observation period of at least 12 h was recommended and ancillary testing was not required when an irreversible cause existed. However, with present ECS or absent CBF, the observation period in this age group could be further decreased.

In AAP 2011 guidelines, although some of the above precautions were revised, especially about the necessity of ancillary studies, there are still special considerations about the term newborns (37 weeks gestation to 30 days of life) in:

- *Clinical examination:* There is a concern about the maturation of brainstem reflexes on this age group and the difficulties arisen with the clinical examination. Therefore, a longer time of 24 h is recommended both before the initial evaluation for BD and for the observation period between tests. In cases of uncertainty, repeated clinical examinations are preferable to ancillary studies.

- *Apnea test:* Particularities of apnea testing in neonates are caused by the possibility that high oxygen pressures during preoxygenation may inhibit the potential stimulation of respiratory centers, and profound bradycardia may precede the gradual development of hypercapnia during apnea. The definition of a valid apnea test is the same as in older children.

- *Ancillary studies:* They are less sensitive in detecting brain electrical activity or cerebral blood flow than in older children. When both ancillary studies were conducted in 149 suspected BD neonates <1 month, absence of CBF (63%), although low, was more sensitive than demonstration of ECS (40%), which was even lower. Disparities were also recorded between studies; when the first examination showed ECS, the absence of CBF was confirmed in 66.7% of patients, while when the absence of flow was firstly recorded, ECS was present in only 42% of patients. Due to limitation of ancillary tests for this age, repeated clinical neurological examinations are indicated than relying on ancillary tests. However, when ancillary tests are present and compatible with BD, the inter-examination interval could be shortened at the same way as happened to older children.

Similar recommendations for patients younger than 36 weeks to 1 month of age were issued by the ANZICS 2013 guidelines as well, stating that the initial evaluation for BD should defer for 48 h, with an interval of 24 h between the two tests [14].

6. Special considerations in patients younger than 2 months by RCCHD 2015 guidelines

Due to uncertainty about the validity of the 2008 AoMRC code of practice DNC criteria in young infants, in the UK, the RCCHD examined literature evidence for BD in very young patients from 37 weeks corrected gestation (postmenstrual) to 2 months postterm [18]. According to their guidelines, DNC is a clinical diagnosis with certain preconditions, and ancillary tests do not help in this diagnosis. They recommended that DNC for this age group should be made taking into account the following:

- *Preconditions:* The same preconditions are recommended as those detailed in the 2008 AoMRC code of practice and in the 1991 BPA report, with an additional prerequisite about the first clinical examination. Postasphyxiated infants or those receiving intensive care after resuscitation, having or not being treated with therapeutic hypothermia, should have a period of at least 24 h of observation. This observation period could be extended in the case of suspected residual drug-induced sedation.

- *Clinical diagnosis of DNC:* The same DNC clinical criteria are recommended as those used in the 2008 AoMRC code of practice for adults, children, and older infants, with special considerations on apnea. A stronger hypercarbic stimulus is used to establish respiratory unresponsiveness. Specifically, there should be a clear rise in $PaCO_2$ levels of >2.7 kPa (>20 mm Hg) *above a baseline of at least 5.3 kPa (40 mm Hg)* to >8.0 kPa (60 mm Hg) with no respiratory response at that level. Two clinical examinations are required with the same interval as in 2008 AoMRC code of practice.

- *Ancillary tests:* Ancillary tests were not found sufficiently robust to help confidently diagnose DNC in infants. They are required only in cases where a clinical diagnosis of DNC is not possible (for example because of extensive faciomaxillary injuries, or high cervical cord injury).

- *Examiners:* Two qualified pediatricians who have been registered for more than 5 years and are competent in the procedure are required. At least one should be a consultant. They should perform successfully two tests, including apnea.

7. Special considerations for premature newborns

Brainstem reflexes are not fully developed in premature babies, for example the pupillary response to light appears at 30 weeks, but is only consistently present at 32–35 weeks of gestation, and the central respiratory response to CO_2 is relatively poorly developed below 33 weeks of gestation. Due to the uncertainty surrounding this issue, there are not any international guidelines to address BD diagnosis in premature babies below 36–37 weeks postconceptual age [14, 20].

8. Declaration of death: documentation

Death is declared after the second neurologic examination and apnea test confirms an unchanged and irreversible condition. When there is a concern about the validity of the first clinical examination and ancillary studies are used, documentation of components from the second clinical examination that can be completed, including a second apnea test, must remain consistent with brain death. Documentation at each step of diagnosis is necessary, starting from the preconditions that should be met and finishing with the exact time of death, accompanied by the well written names and signatures of the responsible physicians. The use of a checklist provides standardized documentation to determine brain death ensuring that no step is missing and is highly recommended [20, 21, 24]. A checklist outlining essential examination and testing components is provided in Appendix 2.

The law, almost worldwide, recognizes that after DB declaration, preservation of technology-dependent life in modern ICUs is of no use, unless the patient is going to be an organ donor, whereas all the necessary actions should be undertaken. Time of clinical death after BD varies in different references according to national social, cultural, and religious preferences. In a preliminary announcement of our study, this time was approximately 2.74 days after the completion of the second apnea test, mainly attributed to the high emotional stress of the parents and the time needed by the family to accept the reality of BD for their children [39]. In one of the first relevant studies in children, it is reported that among 171 BD pediatric patients 47% had their ventilatory support withdrawn an average of 1.7 days after the diagnosis of BD, whereas in 46% support was continued until a cardiac arrest that happened an average of 22.7 days later [40]. The shorter period of 8.52 h is reported in Canada [2] and the longer period up to 4 years is recorded in Japan [7].

9. Parental support

The loss of a child is the most powerful emotional stress for a family. Moreover, there is evidence that parents cannot understand the concept of the brain death in a child that is apparently alive, connecting to ventilator with its heart beating. Good communication between the family and the medical team is necessary to make clear that, despite everything had been made for the recovery of their children, they will have a dismal outcome. The role of the bedside nurse who spent more time with the patients and the parents is fundamental in creating the trust to accept the reality of BD. From the very beginning of the admission of their child at the PICU, the parents should be fully informed of the disease, the treatments and the unfavorable prognosis. When parents are not well informed, they will take longer to understand the evolution to BD and accept the death of their child [7, 23].

Communication with families must be clear and concise, yet using a simple language without pompous medical terminology that they could not understand. Apart medical and nursing team, other medical workers could help families cope with the apparent death as well. The clerk and psychotherapists/psychologists may help them to take difficult end-of-life decisions and parents should be offered this possibility. The presence of family during the tests is questionable. Some families may find it helpful and relieving to see each diagnostic step and the complete loss of responsiveness, but a danger of severe emotional embarrassment lurks in case spinal reflexes are elicited [7]. The family must understand that after the confirmation of BD, their child meets legal criteria for death and continuation of medical therapies, including ventilator support, is no longer an option unless organ donation is planned [20].

10. Conclusions

Diagnosing BD in children is a challenging task and despite the existence of pediatric guidelines since 1987, great variation has been recorded. Strict adherence to published guidelines and medical standards for determining brain death is the minimum requirement for maintaining public trust. The neurological criteria, as outlined above, represent international practice in which the medical profession and the public can have complete confidence [16]. The use of checklist promotes the necessary documentation of each part of declaration of BD and is strongly recommended [2, 21, 24]. International guidelines should form a basis where national guidelines could be established, taking into account legal, ethical, cultural, and religious differences. Diagnosing BD is a medical duty and should be faced with the appropriate knowledge and responsibility.

Although it becomes more and more clear that BD is a clinical diagnosis, there are circumstances where ancillary studies are still necessary. Technology is rapidly evolving and newer methods assessing brain function are developed. Newer methods to assess CBF and neurophysiologic function comparing them to traditional ancillary studies is a forthcoming need, and they will be probably included in future guidelines to assist with determination of brain death in children. Additional information or studies are required to determine if a single neurologic examination is sufficient for neonates, infants, and children to determine brain death as currently recommended for adults over 18 years of age, by the 2010 AAN adult guidelines on BD [12, 20].

Appendices

Appendix 1. Brain death diagnosis algorithm (adapted from Ref. [20])

Appendix 2. Check list for determination of brain death (adapted from Ref. [20])

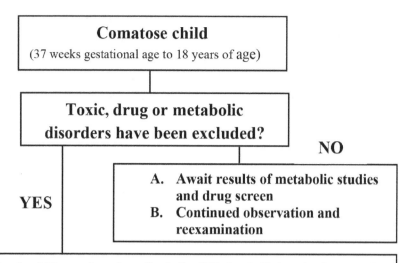

Brain Death Examination for Infants and Children
Two physicians must perform independent examinations separated by specified intervals

Patient name and age	Timing of first exam	Observation period
Term newborn 37 wks gestational age and up to 30 days old	☐ 24h after birth OR following CPR or SBI	☐ At least 24h ☐ Shortened due to ancillary study consistent with BD
31 days to 18 years	☐ 24h after CPR or SBI	☐ At least 12h ☐ Shortened due to ancillary study consistent with BD

Section 1. PRECONDITIONS for brain death examinations and apnea test

A. IRREVERSIBLE AND IDENTIFIABLE CAUSE OF COMA
☐ Traumatic brain injury ☐ Anoxic Brain injury ☐ Known metabolic disorder ☐ Other (specify)

B. CORRECTION OF CONTRIBUTING FACTORS	Examination 1		Examination 2	
a. Core Body Temperature > 35°C	☐ Yes	☐ No	☐ Yes	☐ No
b. Systolic blood pressure or MAP at acceptable range	☐ Yes	☐ No	☐ Yes	☐ No
c. Sedative /analgesic drugs excluded	☐ Yes	☐ No	☐ Yes	☐ No
d. Metabolic intoxication/abnormalities excluded	☐ Yes	☐ No	☐ Yes	☐ No
e. Neuromuscular/antiepileptic drugs excluded	☐ Yes	☐ No	☐ Yes	☐ No

☐ If ALL preconditions are marked YES, then proceed to the next section, OR
☐ .... confounding variable was present. Ancillary study was performed to document BD.

Section 2. PHYSICAL EXAMINATION *Note: Spinal Cord Reflexes are Acceptable*	Examination 1 Date/time:		Examination 2 Date/time:	
a. Flaccid tone, unresponsive to deep painful stimuli	☐ Yes	☐ No	☐ Yes	☐ No
b. Pupils are midpositioned or fully dilated and non reactive	☐ Yes	☐ No	☐ Yes	☐ No
c. Corneal, cough, gag reflexes absent	☐ Yes	☐ No	☐ Yes	☐ No
Sucking and rooting reflexes absent (infants/neonates)	☐ Yes	☐ No	☐ Yes	☐ No
d. Oculovestibular (caloric) reflexes absent	☐ Yes	☐ No	☐ Yes	☐ No
e. Spontaneous respirations on ventilator absent	☐ Yes	☐ No	☐ Yes	☐ No

The .... (specify) element could not be performed because of ....
☐ Ancillary study (EEG or radionuclide CBF) was therefore performed to document BD.

Section 3. APNEA TEST *Aim to baseline eucapnia $PaCO_2 \geq 40$ mm Hg*	Examination 1 Date/Time:	Examination 2 Date/Time:
No spontaneous respiratory efforts were observed despite final $PaCO_2 \geq 60$ mm Hg and a ≥ 20 mm Hg increase above baseline (examinations 1 & 2)	Pretest $PaCO_2$: Apnea (min): Pretest $PaCO_2$:	Pretest $PaCO_2$: Apnea (min): Pretest $PaCO_2$:

Section 4. ANCILLARY TESTING	Date/Time:		
☐ Elecroencephalogram (EEG) report documents electocerebral silence (ECS) OR		☐ Yes	☐ No
☐ Cerebral Blood Flow (CBF) study report documents no cerebral perfusion		☐ Yes	☐ No

Section 5. Signatures

Examiner One
I certify that my examination is consistent with cessation of function of the brain and the brainstem. Confirmatory examination to follow.

(Printed Name)   (Signature)
(Specialty)   (Lisence)   (Date mm/dd/yyyy)   (Time)

Examiner Two
☐ I certify that my examination ☐ and/or ancillary test report ☐ confirms unchanged and irreversible cessation of function of the brain and the brainstem. **The patient is declared dead at this time.**

Date/Time of Death:

(Printed Name)   (Signature)
(Specialty)   (Lisence)   (Date mm/dd/yyyy)   (Time)

CPR; Cardiopulmonary Resuiscitation, SBI; Severe Brain Injury

Author details

Eleni Athanasios Volakli*, Peristera-Eleni Mantzafleri, Serafeia Kalamitsou, Asimina Violaki, Elpis Chochliourou, Menelaos Svirkos, Athanasios Kasimis and Maria Sdougka

*Address all correspondence to: elenavolakli@gmail.com

Pediatric Intensive Care Unit, Hippokration General Hospital, Thessaloniki, Greece

References

[1] Swedish Committee on Defining Death. The Concept of Death. Summary. Stockholm: Swedish Ministry of Health and Social Affairs; 1984. p. 38

[2] Joffe AR, Shemie SD, Farrell C, Hutchison J, McCarthy-Tamblyn L. Brain death in Canadian PICUs: Demographics, timing, and irreversibility. Pediatric Critical Care Medicine. 2013;**14**:1-9

[3] Burns PJ, Sellers ED, Meyer CE, Lewis-Newby S, Truog RD. Epidemiology of death in the pediatric intensive care unit at five U.S. teaching hospitals. Critical Care Medicine. 2014;**42**(9):2101-2108

[4] Lee KJ, Tieves K, Scanlon CM. Alterations in end-of-life support in the pediatric intensive care unit. Pediatrics. 2010;**126**:e859-e864

[5] Volakli AE, Chochliourou E, Dimitriadou M, Violaki A, Mantzafleri P, Samkinidou E, et al. Death analysis in pediatric intensive care patients. Critical Care. 2016;**20**(Suppl 2):P451

[6] Spanish Society of Intensive and Critical Care and Units Coronary. Transplants: Percentage of Patients Diagnosed with Brain Death. NQMC:008518; 2011 March. Available from: http://www.qualitymeasures.ahrq.gov/summaries/summary/43713/...[Accessed: November 10, 2016]

[7] Shemie SD, Pollack MM, Morioka M, Bonner S. Diagnosis of brain death in children. The Lancet Neurology. 2007;**6**(1):87-92

[8] Koszer S, Moshe LS, Kao A, Riviello JJ. Determination of Brain Death in Children [Internet]. Available from: http://www.emedicine.medscape.com/article/1177999-Updated Oct 5, 2016. [Accessed: November 10, 2016]

[9] Ad Hoc Committee of the Harvard Medical School. A definition of irreversible coma. Report of the Ad Hoc Committee of the Harvard Medical School to examine the definition of brain death. The Journal of the American Medical Association. 1968;**205**(6):337-340

[10] President's Commission. Guidelines for the determination of death. Report of the medical consultants on the diagnosis of death to the President's commission for the study of ethical problems in medicine and biomedical and behavioral research. The Journal of the American Medical Association. 1981;**246**(19):2184-2186

[11] Wijdicks FME. Determining brain death in adults. Neurology. 1995;**45**:1003-1011

[12] Wijdicks EFM, Varelas NP, Gronseth SG, Greer MD. Evidence-based guideline update: Determining brain death in adults. Neurology. 2010;**74**:1911-1918

[13] Academy of Medical Royal Colleges. A Code of Practice for the Diagnosis and Confirmation of Death [Internet]. 2008. Available from: http://www.aomrc.org.uk/doc_details/42-a-code-ofpractice-for-the-diagnosis-and-confirmation-of-death [Accessed: January 20, 2017]

[14] Australian and New Zealand Intensive Care Society. The ANZICS Statement on Death and Organ Donation (Edition 3.2). Melbourne: ANZICS; 2013

[15] Shemie SD, Ross H, Pagliarello J, et al. Brain arrest: The neurological determination of death and organ donor management in Canada: Organ donor management in Canada: Recommendations of the forum on medical management to optimize donor organ potential. Canadian Medical Association Journal. 2006;**174**:S13

[16] Gardiner D, Shemie S, Manar A, Opdam H. International perspective on the diagnosis of death. British Journal of Anaesthesia. 2012;**108**(S1):i14-i28. DOI: 10.1093/bja/aer397

[17] British Paediatric Association. Diagnosis of brain stem death in children. A Working Party Report; 1991

[18] Marikar D. The diagnosis of death by neurological criteria in infants less than 2 months old: RCPCH guideline 2015. Archives of Disease in Childhood Education and Practice Edition. 2016;**101**(4):186. DOI: 10.1136/archdischild-2015-309706. Epub 2016 Mar 9

[19] Task Force for the Determination of Brain Death in Children. Guidelines for the determination of brain death in children. Task force for the determination of brain death in children. Archives of Neurology. 1987;**44**(6):587-588

[20] Thomas A. Nakagawa, Stephen Ashwal, Mudit Mathur, Mohan Mysore, and the society of critical care medicine, section on critical care and section on neurology of the american academy of pediatrics, and the child neurology society. Clinical report—Guidelines for the determination of brain death in infants and children: An update of the 1987 Task Force recommendations. Pediatrics. 2011;**128**:e720-e740

[21] Mathur M, Petersen LC, Stadtler M, Rose C, Ejike JC, Petersen F, et al. Variability in pediatric brain death determination and documentation in Southern California. Pediatrics. 2008;**121**:988

[22] Wijdicks EFM, Rabinstein AA, Manno ME, et al. Pronouncing brain death: Contemporary practice and safety of the apnea test. Neurology. 2008;**71**:1240

[23] Paul B. Diagnosis and management of brain death in children. Current Paediatrics. 2005;**15**:301-307

[24] Shore PM. Following guidelines for brain death examinations: A matter of trust. Pediatric Critical Care Medicine. 2013;**14**:98-99. DOI: 10.1097/PCC.0b013e31826775bb

[25] Zielinski PB. Brain death, the pediatric patient, and the nurse. Pediatric Nursing. 2011;**37**(1):17-21

[26] Kochanek PM, Carney N, Adelson PD, et al. American Academy of Pediatrics-Section on Neurological Surgery; American Association of Neurological Surgeons/Congress of Neurological Surgeons; Child Neurology Society; European Society of Pediatric and Neonatal Intensive Care; Neurocritical Care Society; Pediatric Neurocritical Care Research Group; Society of Critical Care Medicine; Paediatric Intensive Care Society UK; Society for Neuroscience in Anesthesiology and Critical Care; World Federation of Pediatric Intensive and Critical Care Societies. Guidelines for the acute medical management of severe traumatic brain injury in infants, children, and adolescents. Pediatric Critical Care Medicine. 2012;**13** Suppl 1:S1-S82. DOI: 10.1097/PCC.0b013e31823f437e

[27] Practical procedures: Airway and breathing. In: Samuels M, Wieteska S, editors. Advanced Pediatric Life Support. 5th ed. Wiley-Blackwell, Atrium, Southern Gate, Chichester, West Sussex, UK; 2010. pp. 210-211

[28] La Mancusa J, Cooper R, Vieth R, Wright F. The effects of the falling therapeutic and sub-therapeutic barbiturate blood levels on electrocerebral silence in clinically brain-dead children. Clinical Electroencephalography. 1991;**22**(2):112-117

[29] JScott JB, Gentile AM, Bennett NS, Couture MA, MacIntyre RN. Apnea testing during Brain Death Assessment: A review of clinical practice and published literature. Respiratory Care. 2013;**58**(3):532-538

[30] Outwaker KM, Rockoff MA. Apnea testing to confirm brain death in children. Critical Care Medicine. 1984;**12**(4):357-358

[31] Rowland TW, Donnelly JH, Jackson AH. Apnea documentation for determination of brain death in children. Pediatrics. 1984;**74**(4):505-508

[32] Riviello JJ, Sapin JI, Brown LW, et al. Hypoxemia and hemodynamic changes during the hypercarbia stimulation test. Pediatric Neurology. 1988;**4**(4):213-218

[33] Paret G, Barzilay Z. Apnea testing in suspected brain dead children: Physiological and mathematical modeling. Intensive Care Medicine. 1995;**21**(3):247-252

[34] Vardis R, Pollack MM. Altered apnea threshold in a pediatric patient with suspected brain death. Critical Care Medicine. 1998;**26**(11):1917-1919

[35] Brilli RJ, Bigos D. Threshold in a child with suspected brain death. Journal of Child Neurology. 1995;**10**(3):245-246

[36] Schafer JA, Caronna JJ. Duration of apnea needed to confirm brain death. Neurology. 1978;**28**:661

[37] Bar-Joseph G, Bar-Lavie Y, Zonis Z. Tension pneumothorax during apnea testing for the determination of brain death. Anesthesiology. 1998;**89**(5):1250-1251

[38] Burns JD, Russell JA. Tension pneumothorax complicating apnea testing during brain death evaluation. Journal of Clinical Neuroscience. 2008;**15**(5):580-582

[39] Mantzafleri PE, Volakli E, Violakli A, Chochliourou E, Svirkos M, Kasimis A, et al. Incidence and management of brain death in a Greek PICU. European Journal of Pediatrics. 2016;**175**(11):1393-1880:E-poster 1105

[40] Ashwal S, Schneider S. Brain death in children: Part I. Pediatric Neurology. 1987;**3**(1):5-11

Permissions

All chapters in this book were first published in CTICM&IC, by InTech Open; hereby published with permission under the Creative Commons Attribution License or equivalent. Every chapter published in this book has been scrutinized by our experts. Their significance has been extensively debated. The topics covered herein carry significant findings which will fuel the growth of the discipline. They may even be implemented as practical applications or may be referred to as a beginning point for another development.

The contributors of this book come from diverse backgrounds, making this book a truly international effort. This book will bring forth new frontiers with its revolutionizing research information and detailed analysis of the nascent developments around the world.

We would like to thank all the contributing authors for lending their expertise to make the book truly unique. They have played a crucial role in the development of this book. Without their invaluable contributions this book wouldn't have been possible. They have made vital efforts to compile up to date information on the varied aspects of this subject to make this book a valuable addition to the collection of many professionals and students.

This book was conceptualized with the vision of imparting up-to-date information and advanced data in this field. To ensure the same, a matchless editorial board was set up. Every individual on the board went through rigorous rounds of assessment to prove their worth. After which they invested a large part of their time researching and compiling the most relevant data for our readers.

The editorial board has been involved in producing this book since its inception. They have spent rigorous hours researching and exploring the diverse topics which have resulted in the successful publishing of this book. They have passed on their knowledge of decades through this book. To expedite this challenging task, the publisher supported the team at every step. A small team of assistant editors was also appointed to further simplify the editing procedure and attain best results for the readers.

Apart from the editorial board, the designing team has also invested a significant amount of their time in understanding the subject and creating the most relevant covers. They scrutinized every image to scout for the most suitable representation of the subject and create an appropriate cover for the book.

The publishing team has been an ardent support to the editorial, designing and production team. Their endless efforts to recruit the best for this project, has resulted in the accomplishment of this book. They are a veteran in the field of academics and their pool of knowledge is as vast as their experience in printing. Their expertise and guidance has proved useful at every step. Their uncompromising quality standards have made this book an exceptional effort. Their encouragement from time to time has been an inspiration for everyone.

The publisher and the editorial board hope that this book will prove to be a valuable piece of knowledge for researchers, students, practitioners and scholars across the globe.

List of Contributors

Bogdan Pavel
Division of Physiology and Neurosciences, University of Medicine and Pharmacy "Carol Davila", Bucharest, Romania
Emergency Hospital Plastic Surgery and Burns, Bucharest, Romania

Selim Öncel
Division of Pediatric Infectious Diseases, Department of Pediatrics and Child Health, Section of Internal Medical Sciences, Kocaeli University Faculty of Medicine, Kocaeli, Turkey

Muntean Delia and Licker Monica
"Victor Babes" University of Medicine and Pharmacy, Timisoara, Romania

Faustino J. Renteria
Intensive Care Unit, Hospital Español, Mexico City, Mexico

Jose J. Zaragoza
Intensive Care Unit, Hospital Español, Mexico City, Mexico
Mexican College of Critical Care Medicine, Mexico City, Mexico

Dyah Kanya Wati
Critical Care Medicine, Udayana University Sanglah Hospital, Denpasar, Bali, Indonesia

Zsolt Bodnar
Letterkenny University Hospital, Letterkenny, Ireland

Maribel Ibarra-Sarlat, Graciela Castañeda-Muciño and Juan Carlos Núñez-Enríquez
UMAE Hospital de Pediatría Centro Médico Nacional Siglo XXI, Instituto Mexicano del Seguro Social, México City, Mexico

Eduardo Terrones-Vargas
Unidad de Cuidados Intensivos Pediátricos, Hospital Infantil de México Federico Gómez, Secretaria de Salud, México City, Mexico

Lizett Romero-Espinoza
UMAE Hospital Gineco-Obstetricia No.3 "Dr. Victor Manuel Espinosa De Los Reyes Sánchez", Centro Médico Nacional La Raza, Mexico City, Mexico

Alejandro Herrera-Landero
Hospital de Traumatología y Ortopedia «Lomas Verdes», Instituto Mexicano del Seguro Social, State of Mexico, Mexico

Nabil Abdelhamid Shallik
Hamad Medical Corporation, Clinical Anesthesiology, Weill Cornell Medical College in Qatar, Doha, Qatar
Anesthesia and ICU Department, Tanta Faculty of Medicine, Tanta, Egypt
Anesthesia Section of Rumailah Hospital, Anesthesia, ICU and Perioperative Medicine Department HMC, Doha, Qatar
Medical Education and Qatar Robotic Surgery Center, HMC, Doha, Qatar

Mamdouh Almustafa and Ahmed Zaghw
Department of Anesthesia, ICU and Perioperative Medicine, HMC, Doha, Qatar

Abbas Moustafa
Elminia University, Egypt
Radiology, HMC, Doha, Qatar

Eleni Athanasios Volakli, Peristera-Eleni Mantzafleri, Serafeia Kalamitsou, Asimina Violaki, Elpis Chochliourou, Menelaos Svirkos, Athanasios Kasimis and Maria Sdougka
Pediatric Intensive Care Unit, Hippokration General Hospital, Thessaloniki, Greece

Index

A
Abdominal Compartment Syndrome, 93-95, 104
Acute Kidney Injury, 69-70, 79-82, 90
Acute Renal Failure, 30, 69, 79-82
Acute Tubular Necrosis, 32, 70-71, 82
Anesthesia, 1-3, 5-19, 21, 23, 125-126, 129-130, 132, 138-140, 151, 156-157, 159, 171
Apnea Testing, 160, 162, 164-166, 169-172, 174-176, 184-185

B
Bispectral Index, 2, 7, 11, 16-19, 174
Blood Pressure, 23-24, 36-37, 87-88, 107, 132, 170-171
Body Mass Index, 130, 145
Brain Death, 160-162, 166-168, 170, 172-175, 178-179, 182-185
Brainstem Reflexes, 160-161, 163, 166, 168, 172, 176-177
Bronchoscopy, 49, 128, 140-143, 145-147, 152, 159
Burst Suppression, 1-3, 14-16

C
Central Venous Saturation, 87
Cerebral Oximetry Monitoring, 2, 20
Consciousness Index, 9
Continuous Intra-abdominal Pressure Monitoring, 93, 95, 98, 102-103
Cortical Connectivity, 1-2, 12-13, 15, 21
Cortical Reactivity, 1, 9, 14, 20-21
Corticosteroids, 22, 39
Creatinine, 24, 70-71, 74, 76, 79, 81
Crystalloids, 36, 86
Cystatin C, 74, 81

D
Diffuse Axonal Injury, 3

E
Electroencephalographic, 1, 5, 10, 14-16, 18
Endotracheal Intubation, 49, 105-107, 124-126, 131, 142, 155, 157
Entropy, 1, 6-7, 9-10, 12, 16-19

F
Flexible Fiberoptic Intubation, 128, 137
Fluid Management, 83, 85-88, 91-92
Fluid Resuscitation, 33, 36, 45, 83, 87, 90-91

G
Glomerular Filtration Rate, 32, 69-70, 81

H
Hypercarbia, 106, 184
Hypovolemia, 52, 72, 87-88, 130
Hypoxia, 3, 20, 29, 31, 36, 40, 53, 73, 106, 129, 151, 164, 169-172

I
Intra-abdominal Hypertension, 93, 95, 103-104
Intra-abdominal Pressure, 93-98, 102-104
Intracranial Pressure, 11, 19, 94, 161, 163
Intravascular Volume, 69, 76, 83-84, 86-87
Ischemia-reperfusion Injury, 70, 73

L
Linezolid, 51, 60-61, 63
Listeria Monocytogenes, 22, 25

M
Macrolide, 38, 51
MAP, 87-88
Microvascular Dysfunction, 89
Midazolam, 9, 13, 21, 111, 140, 163

N
Near-infrared Spectroscopy, 2, 11, 20
Neonatal Sepsis, 22, 30, 43
Noxious Stimuli, 1-2, 168

P
P. Aeruginosa, 50, 53, 57, 60-61
Paralytic Ileus, 93-94
Pediatric Intensive Care Unit, 45, 83, 90, 127, 160-161, 182
Permutation Entropy, 1, 10, 18-19
Pneumonia, 39, 46, 48-50, 63, 66-67, 138, 142

Pneumothorax, 38, 94, 114, 142, 144, 155, 158, 185
Prerenal Aki, 69, 71-72, 76

R
Raas, 72, 84
Rapid Sequence Intubation, 105, 107, 110, 122-124, 130
Renal Dysfunction, 24, 167
Renal Replacement Therapy, 69-71, 77, 81-82, 84, 89
Respiratory Dysfunction, 24

S
Sepsis, 22-23, 25-36, 38-49, 52-53, 63, 67-68, 70-71, 73-74, 79-80, 84-91
Septic Shock, 22-23, 25-26, 28-31, 33-34, 36, 39-43, 45-48, 53, 68, 73, 84, 86, 88, 90-92, 111
Severe Trauma, 105
Spectral Edge Frequency, 6, 9, 15-16, 18
Succinylcholine, 111, 130-131

Systemic Inflammatory Response Syndrome, 22-23, 44

T
Tracheal Intubation, 116, 125, 127-130, 132-133, 157
Tracheal Stenosis, 143-144, 158
Tracheostomy, 49, 128, 138, 141-146, 150-151, 155, 158-159, 170
Tracheostomy Tube, 141-142, 144-146
Traumatic Brain Injury, 1, 8, 14, 20-21, 166, 184

U
Urinary Catheter, 93

V
Vancomycin, 38-39, 51, 53, 57-61, 63
Videolaryngoscopy, 126, 128, 132-133, 135-137
Virtual Endoscopy, 128, 152
Visceral Oedema, 93-94

CPSIA information can be obtained
at www.ICGtesting.com
Printed in the USA
BVHW011734220519
549014BV00003B/357/P